TRADITIONAL MEDICINES
AROUND THE WORLD

Matthew N. O. Sadiku
Janet O. Sadiku
Sarhan M. Musa

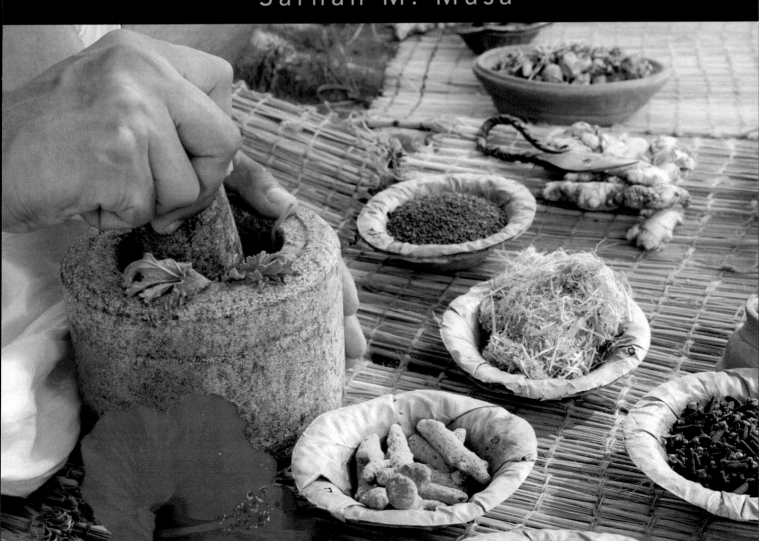

Traditional Medicines Around The World

iUniverse books may be ordered through booksellers or by contacting:

iUniverse
1663 Liberty Drive
Bloomington, IN 47403
www.iuniverse.com
844-349-9409

ISBN: 978-1-6632-3838-2 (sc)
ISBN: 978-1-6632-3836-8 (hc)
ISBN: 978-1-6632-3837-5 (e)

Library of Congress Control Number: 2022906845

Print information available on the last page.

iUniverse rev. date: 05/18/2022

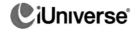

Dedicated to our parents:

Ayisat and Solomon Sadiku
John and Esther Babafemi
Fatimeh and Mahmoud Musa

BRIEF TABLE OF CONTENTS

1. Introduction 1

2. Traditional Chinese Medicine 20

3. Traditional Indian Medicine 36

4. Japanese Traditional Medicine 54

5. European Traditional Medicine 70

6. African Traditional Medicine 83

7. Yoruba Traditional Medicine 101

8. Persian Traditional Medicine 119

9. Traditional Arabic and Islamic Medicine 134

10. Mexician Traditonal Medicine 150

11. Traditional Mediterranean Diet 166

12. Future of Traditional Medicine...184

    Appendix A – Other Traditional Medicines........................199

    Index 201

DISCLAIMER

The information in this book is for enlightenment purposes only and should not be used as a replacement for professional diagnosis and treatments. No content on this book should ever be used as a substitute for direct medical advice from your doctor or other qualified clinician. Always consult your healthcare provider before making any health-related decisions.

PREFACE

Our health is our most important asset. Health and the provision of healthcare is fundamental to the welfare of any nation. It has been well said that "a healthy man is a wealthy man." In spite of advances in science and medicine, disease remains a serious threat to public health in both developed and developing nations. The desire to have and sustain good health cuts across national, cultural, geographic, and political boundaries.

Every region of the world has had one form of traditional medicine at some stage in its history. Traditional medicines have been a part of human history all over the world, with knowledge being transferred from generation to generation. The knowledge of traditional medicine is increasingly drawing attention worldwide due to its significant role in meeting the global public health needs.

Folk or traditional medicine (TM) refers to diverse health practices, knowledge, and skills based on ancient indigenous experience that are used to maintain health as well as to cure, diagnose, or prevent illness. TM is also known as "complementary," "alternative" or "non-conventional" medicine. It is a major foundation on which modern medicine has been built. It is called traditional for a reason: it is old fashioned. It refers to the combination of indigenous practices of medicine and several therapeutic experiences of previous generations for the treatment, control, and management of illnesses. It entails health practices, approaches, knowledge, and beliefs incorporating plant, animal, mineral based medicines, spiritual therapies, manual techniques, diagnose, and preventing illnesses or maintaining well-being. TM has been used to cure many diseases including skin diseases, tuberculosis, diabetes, jaundice, hypertension, mental disorders, cancer, cardiovascular care, erectile dysfunction, HIV, and AIDS. The use of traditional medicine for health purposes has increased in both developing and developed countries. It is still generally available, affordable, and commonly used in large parts of Africa, Asia, and Latin America. For this reason, the World Health Organization (WHO) is encouraging the integration of traditional medicine into Western medicine. The two systems of medicine can be complementary, each strengthening the inadequacies of the other.

This book focuses on ten most popular traditional medicines around the world. The book is organized into 12 chapters. The first chapter provides an introduction to the practice of traditional medicine all over the world. It serves as an introduction to the book. Chapter 2 covers the traditional Chinese medicine (TCM), which is perhaps the most popular and well-research traditional medicine. It is one of the acknowledged natural medicines classified by WHO. Some of its precepts were standardized in the People's Republic of China, where the government promoted a systematized form of TCM. Chapter 3 provides an overview of the traditional Indian medicine. India is blessed with an ancient heritage of traditional Indian medicine (TIM), which relies on lifelong medication on which patients can depend. TIM remains one of the most ancient yet living traditions. The chapter considers the six India traditional medicinal systems and focusses on the most popular system, Ayurveda.

In chapter 4, we cover the Japanese traditional medicine, Kampo, which is a holistic and individualized treatment with a long tradition. Kampo is a diverse and dynamic form of medicine. Perhaps the most interesting aspect of Japanese medicine is the rapidity with which it became Westernized and scientific. Chapter 5 addresses European traditional medicine, which essentially refers to traditional therapies that have their origin in Europe and is practiced throughout the European Union. Although Europe remains to be a leader in herbal medicine, European traditional medicine is currently in a state of decline. Chapter 6 deals with African traditional medicine, which is a holistic healthcare system that has three components or levels of specialty: divination, spiritualism, and herbalism. Traditional African medicine refers to indigenous forms of healing that are practiced all over the continent of Africa. It is regarded as the oldest of all therapeutic systems.

While chapter 6 deals with the general African medicine, Chapter 7 focuses on a specific, popular African medicine, the Yoruba traditional medicine. The Yorùbá people of southwestern Nigeria are one of the most researched ethno-linguistic groups in Africa. They have an impressive system of indigenous medicine. For the Yoruba, reality is rooted in both the physical and the spiritual realms. Chapter 8 presents

Persian traditional medicine, which is a set of knowledge and skills in the diagnosis, prevention, and treatment of diseases from ancient times till now. Iran is formerly known as Persia. Iranian traditional medicine (also known as Persian medicine) is one of famous forms of traditional medicine. Iranians have always relied on their traditional medicines to treat various diseases. Chapter 9 addresses Traditional Arabic Islamic Medicine, which evolved from Graeco-Roman, Chinese, Persian, and Ayurvedic medical practices. It was developed in medieval times and practiced in various Arabic countries today. It is the system of healing practiced since antiquity in the Arab world with the influence of Islam. TAIM incorporates herbal medicines, spiritual therapies, dietary practices, and manual techniques.

In chapter 10, we address Mexican traditional medicine, which consists of Mexican healing practices that have survived conquest, colonization, and modern medicine. The Mexican culture is rich with traditions that are well documented to have existed long before Columbus sailed the ocean blue. Mexico is regarded for its cultural and biological diversity, which is reflected in the vast traditional knowledge of herbal remedies. Chapter 11 covers Traditional Mediterranean diet (MedDiet), which is the old way of eating. It is one of the most studied and well-known dietary models worldwide. The Mediterranean diet has been characterized as the gold standard of diets. It is a pattern of eating that is modeled after the traditional cuisines of nations bordering the Mediterranean Sea. Chapter 12 is the last chapter. It addresses the possible futures of traditional herbal medicines. Traditional medicine needs to be officially legalized and made part of the mainstream healthcare system in every country. The integration of traditional medicine and modern practice will bring about a controlled practice, more responsible, and well harmonized medicine and collaboration among healthcare practitioners. Other traditional medicines not covered in this book are listed in Appendix A.

In a nutshell, this book provides an easy-to-read overview of various traditional medicine across the world. It is a valuable source of guidance for organizations and individuals interested in traditional medicine. The book fills an important niche for medicine. It is a comprehensive, jargon-free introductory text on the healing practices, efficacy, benefits, challenges, and applications of traditional medicine. It provides an introduction to traditional medicine so that beginners can understand TM, its increasing importance, and its developments in contemporary time. It is a must-read book for anyone who cares about traditional. We would like to thank Dr. Pamela Obiomon, dean of College of Engineering at Prairie View A&M University, Texas, for her support.

DETAILED TABLE OF CONTENTS

Chapter 1 – Introduction..1

1.1 Introduction 1

1.2 Brief History Of Medicine 3

1.3 Different Medical Systems 3

1.4 Concept Of Traditional Medicines 6

1.5 Traditional Medicines Around The World..7

1.6 Traditional Herbs...9

1.7 Applications Of Traditional Medicine 12

1.8 Benefits 13

1.9 Challenges 14

1.10 Global Need Of Traditional Medicine 16

1.11 Orgnizations Supporting Tm 16

1.12 Conclusion 17

References...18

Chapter 2 – Traditional Chinese Medicine 20

2.1 Introduction 20

2.2 Brief History Of Tcm...21

2.3 Underlying Concepts 22

2.4 Eight Principles Of Diagnosis 24

2.5 Herbal Medicine 25

2.6 Applications...26

2.7 Modernization...28

2.8 Benefits 29

2.9 Challenges 30

2.10 Conclusion 32

References...33

Chapter 3 – Traditional Indian Medicine 36

3.1 Introduction 36

3.2 Brief History Of Ayurveda...37

3.3 Indian Traditional Medicinal Systems 37

3.4 Ayurvedic System 40

3.5 Herbal Medicine 42

3.6 Applications 44

3.7 Globalization Of Ayurveda 45

3.8 Benefits 47

3.9 Challenges 48

3.10 Conclusion 50

References 51

Chapter 4 – Japanese Traditional Medicine 54

4.1 Introduction 54

4.2 Brief History Of Kampo 55

4.3 Concept Of Japanese Traditional Medicine 55

4.4 Kampo Diagnosis And Treatment 58

4.5 Japanese Herbs 59

4.6 Applications Of Japanese Traditional Medicine 61

4.7 Benefits 64

4.8 Challenges 66

4.9 Taking Kampo Global 66

4.10 Conclusion 67

References 67

Chapter 5 – European Traditional Medicine 70

5.1 Introduction 70

5.2 Brief History Of Etm 71

5.3 Concept Of European Traditional Medicine 71

5.4 European Herbal Medicines 73

5.5 Applications Of Etm 75

5.6 Globalization Of Etm 76

5.7 Benefits 77

5.8 Challenges 77

5.9 Conclusion 80

References 80

Chapter 6 – African Traditional Medicine 83

6.1 Introduction 83

6.2 Brief History Of Atm 84

6.3 Concept Of African Tranditional Medicine 84

6.4 Components Of Atm 85

6.5 Herbal Medicine 86

6.6 Traditional Medicine From Selected Nations 89

6.7 Regulation Of Tradional Medicine 91

6.8 Applications Of Atm 91

6.9 Traditional And Modern Medicine..92

6.10 Benefits..94

6.11 Challenges..94

6.12 Globalization Of Atm..97

6.13 Conclusion..97

References..98

Chapter 7 – Yoruba Traditional Medicine..101

7.1 Introduction..101

1.2 Brief History Of Yoruba Medicine..102

7.3 Concept Of Yoruba Medicine..103

7.4 Yoruba Herbs..105

7.5 Applications Of Yoruba Medicine..108

7.6 Benefits..110

7.7 Challenges..112

7.8 Globalization Of Yoruba Medicine..115

7.9 Conclusion..115

References..116

Chapter 8 – Persian Traditional Medicine..119

8.1 Introduction..119

8.2 Brief History Of Persian Medicine..120

8.3 Concept Of Persian Traditional Medicine..120

8.4 Iranian Herbs..123

8.5 Applications Of Persian Traditional Medicine..126

8.6 Benefits..128

8.7 Challenges..129

8.8 Globalization Of Persian Medicine..129

8.9 Conclusion..130

References..131

Chapter 9 – Traditional Arabic and Islamic Medicine..134

9.1 Introduction..134

9.2 Brief History Of Arabic Medicine..136

9.3 Concept Of Arabic Traditional Medicine..137

9.4 Arabic Herbs..139

9.5 Arabic Medicine In Muslim Nations..142

9.6 Applications Of Arabic Traditional Medicine..143

9.7 Benefits..144

9.8 Challenges..145

9.9 Globalization Of Arabic Medicine..146

9.10 Conclusion..147

References..147

Chapter 10 – Mexician Traditonal Medicine 150

10.1 Introduction 150

10.2 Brief History Of Mexican Medicine 152

10.3 Concept Of Mexican Traditional Medicine 152

10.4 Mexican Herbs 154

10.5 Applications Of Mexican Traditional Medicine 157

10.6 Benefits 158

10.7 Challenges 159

10.9 Globalization Of Mexican Medicine 161

10.9 Conclusion 162

References 163

Chapter 11 – Traditional Mediterranean Diet 166

11.1 Introduction 166

11.2 Brief History Of Meditarian Diet 167

11.3 Mediterranean Herbs 168

11.4 Mediterranean Diet 169

11.5 Other Types Of Mediterranean Diets 173

11.6 Applications Of Mediterranean Diet 174

11.7 Benefits 176

11.8 Challenges 178

11.9 Globalization Of Mediterranean Diet 179

11.10 Conclusion 179

References 180

Chapter 12 – Future of Traditional Medicine 184

12.1 Introduction 184

12.2 Future Of Herbs 185

12.3 Future Of Traditional Medicine 187

12.4 Benefits 189

12.5 Challenges 191

12.6 Globalization Of Traditional Medicine 193

12.7 Modern Technologies 194

12.8 Conclusion 195

References 195

Appendix A – Other Traditional Medicines 199

Index 201

ABOUT THE AUTHORS

A. **Matthew N. O. Sadiku** received his B. Sc. degree in 1978 from Ahmadu Bello University, Zaria, Nigeria, and his M.Sc. and Ph.D. degrees from Tennessee Technological University, Cookeville, TN in 1982 and 1984 respectively. From 1984 to 1988, he was an assistant professor at Florida Atlantic University, Boca Raton, FL, where he did graduate work in computer science. From 1988 to 2000, he was at Temple University, Philadelphia, PA, where he became a full professor. From 2000 to 2002, he was with Lucent/Avaya, Holmdel, NJ as a system engineer and with Boeing Satellite Systems, Los Angeles, CA as a senior scientist. He is presently a professor emeritus of electrical and computer engineering at Prairie View A&M University, Prairie View, TX.

He is the author of over 980 professional papers and over 95 books including *Elements of Electromagnetics* (Oxford University Press, 7th ed., 2018), *Fundamentals of Electric Circuits* (McGraw-Hill, 7th ed., 2021, with C. Alexander), *Computational Electromagnetics with MATLAB* (CRC Press, 4th ed., 2019), *Principles of Modern Communication Systems* (Cambridge University Press, 2017, with S. O. Agbo), and *Emerging Internet-based Technologies* (CRC Press, 2019). In addition to the engineering books, he has written Christian books including *Secrets of Successful Marriages*, *How to Discover God's Will for Your Life*, and commentaries on all the books of the New Testament Bible. Some of his books have been translated into French, Korean, Chinese (and Chinese Long Form in Taiwan), Italian, Portuguese, and Spanish.

He was the recipient of the 2000 McGraw-Hill/Jacob Millman Award for outstanding contributions in the field of electrical engineering. He was also the recipient of the Regents Professor award for 2012-2013 by the Texas A&M University System. He is a registered professional engineer and a fellow of the Institute of Electrical and Electronics Engineers (IEEE) "for contributions to computational electromagnetics and engineering education." He was the IEEE Region 2 Student Activities Committee Chairman. He was an associate editor for IEEE Transactions on Education. He is also a member of the Association for Computing Machinery (ACM) and the American Society of Engineering Education (ASEE). His current research interests are in the areas of computational electromagnetic, computer networks, and engineering education. His works can be found in his autobiography, *My Life and Work* (Trafford Publishing, 2017) or his website: www.matthew-sadiku.com. He currently resides in West Palm Beach, Florida with his wife Janet He can be reached via email at sadiku@ieee.org

B. **Janet O. Sadiku** studied nursing science from 1975 to 1980 at the University of Ife, now known as Obafemi Awolowo University, Nigeria. She has worked as a nurse, educator, and church minister in Nigeria, United Kingdom, and Canada. She is presently retired with her husband in West Palm Beach, FL.

C. **Sarhan M. Musa,** is a professor in Electrical and Computer Engineering Department at Prairie View A&M University. He holds a Ph.D. in Electrical Engineering from the City University of New York.

He is the founder and director of Prairie View Networking Academy (PVNA), Texas. He is LTD Sprint and Boeing Welliver Fellow. Professor Musa is internationally known through his research, scholarly work, and his published books. He has had a number of invited talks at international conferences. He has received a number of prestigious national and university awards and research grants. He is a senior member of the *IEEE* and has also served as a member of the technical program committee and steering committee for a number of major journals and conferences. Professor Musa has written more than a dozen books on various areas in Electrical and Computer Engineering. His current research interests cover many topics in artificial intelligence/machine learning, data analytics, Internet of things, wireless network, data center protocols, renewable energy, power system, and computational methods.

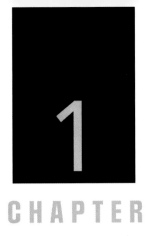

CHAPTER

Introduction

"Let food be thy medicine and medicine be thy food" -Hippocrates

1.1 INTRODUCTION

Health and the provision of healthcare is fundamental to the welfare of any nation. It has been well said that "a healthy man is a wealthy man." Since the dawn of mankind, diseases have been a leading cause of mortality and people have been taking medicines to fight illness or to feel better when they are sick. Humans have used natural products, such as plants, animals, and microorganisms in medicines to alleviate and treat diseases.

In spite of advances in science and medicine, disease remains a serious threat to public health in both developed and developing nations. In recent years, herbs are staging a comeback and herbal "renaissance" occurs all over the world. There has been a resurgence of the use of herbs due to lack of modern therapies for several chronic diseases. This is evident in the increasing number of people worldwide who have been choosing herbal medicines or products to improve their health conditions in recent years [1]. Figure 1.1 shows different health conditions.

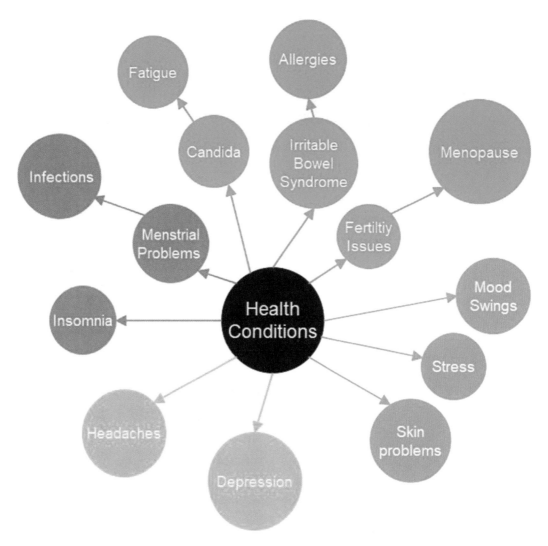

Figure 1.1 Different health conditions.

Tradition medicine (TM) is called traditional for a reason: it is old fashioned. It refers to the combination of indigenous practices of medicine and several therapeutic experiences of many previous generations for the treatment, control, and management of illnesses. TM was the fundamental method used by humans to preserve health and avoid diseases since ancient times.

Traditional medication essentially entails the use of herbal remedies, animal parts, and minerals. It includes a diversity of health practices, approaches, knowledge, spiritual therapies, manual techniques, and exercises, applied to maintain well-being through treating, diagnosing, or preventing illnesses. It is based on a belief that health is a state of balance between several opposing aspects in the human body.. Although modern medicine may exist side-by-side with TM, herbal medicines have often maintained their popularity for historical and cultural reasons [3].

Traditional medicine is often called traditional, conventional, or mainstream. Western medicine. Although traditional medicine is usually community based, it has been used in many countries throughout the world over many centuries. Traditional medicine continues to play an important role worldwide, especially in developing countries. It is widely practiced partly as a supplement and partly as an alternative to modern medicine.

This chapter provides an introduction to the practice of traditional medicine all over the world. It serves as an introduction to the book. It begins by covering different medicine systems. It explains the concept of traditional medicine. It presents traditional medicines and herbs around the world. It covers how traditional medicine is being used by communities around the world. It highlights the benefits and challenges of traditional medicine. It considers the global need of traditional medicine. It mentions the international organizations promoting traditional medicines. The last section concludes with comments.

1.2 BRIEF HISTORY OF MEDICINE

A brief discussion of the history of the use of traditional medicines is provided here. TM has a long history of evolution in practice worldwide and contemporary relevance. The use herbs for healing pave the way for human history and establishes the origin of much modern medicine.

Western medicine (WM) originates from Middle-Eastern and Mediterranean medicine during the Egyptian, Greek, and Roman empires. Back then, the explanation and treatment of all sorts of diseases was based on sacred and spiritual beliefs. WM has established itself as the reference in most nations with undisputable benefits.. It uses healing practices based on scientific evidence and research. Traditional medicine (TM) precedes modern medicine and has a long history. TM is the oldest form of healthcare in the world and is used in the prevention as well as treatment of physical and mental illnesses [4].

Modern medicine was largely disseminated across the world during recent centuries by explorers, missionaries, and merchants. Trade routes linked the Indus valley civilization to Persia, Mesopotamia, and the Arabian Sea. The medieval Islamic world produced some of the greatest medical thinkers in history. They made advances in surgery, built hospitals, and welcomed women into the medical profession. Religion, ethics, and science all came together to produce one of the most fruitful eras in the history of medicine.

China has a long reputation of treating a wide variety of diseases by herbal medicine. This type of medical practice dates back at least 2000 years. Several medical books were published between 100BC to 1900AD. Traditional Chinese medicine emphasizes a holistic approach and focuses on prevention as well as treatment of illness. Chinese immigrants began practicing traditional Chinese medicine in the United States in the 1820s. The use of traditional medicines in the United States declined in the 1940s but returned to popularity in the 1980s.

1.3 DIFFERENT MEDICAL SYSTEMS

Many nations have medical practices described as traditional or folk medicine which may coexist with science-based, institutionalized systems represented by conventional medicine. Thanks to global commercialization and information exchange, patients increasingly have the choice between different medicinal systems for their health care needs. Figure 1.2 shows development of major traditional medicinal systems [5]. To avoid some misunderstanding, it is expedient that we define the following medical concepts [6,7]:

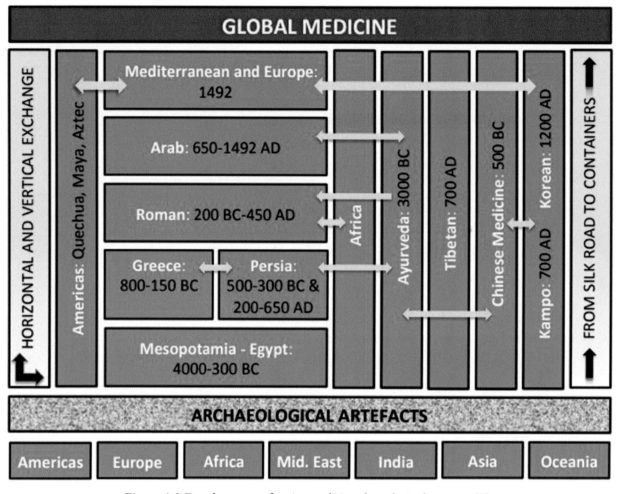

Figure 1.2 Development of major traditional medicinal systems [5].

- *Western Medicine:* The conventional Western medicine evolved in the context of Western and Mediterranean cultures during the Egyptian, Greek, and Roman empires. Modern Western medicine (also referred to as allopathic medicine or scientific medicine) is a system in which health professionals who hold an M.D. (medical doctor) prescribes treatments for specific diseases using drugs, radiation, or surgery. In traditional medicines, healing of patients involves a combination of prayers, magic practices, and herbal mixtures. Western and traditional medicines are based on distinct conceptions of health and disease.

- *Traditional Medicine:* A medical system is regarded "traditional" when it is practiced within the country of origin. According to the World Health Organization, TM is the sum total of the knowledge, skill, and practices based on the theories, beliefs, and experiences indigenous to different cultures, used in the maintenance of health, as well as in the prevention, diagnosis, improvement or treatment of physical and mental illness. The most widely used traditional medicine systems today include those of China, India, Latin America, the Middle East, and Africa. About 80% of Asian and African populations use traditional medicine (TM) to meet their primary healthcare needs.

- *Integrative Medicine:* Integration of TM and modern medicine has been recommended by the WHO since 1978. Integrative medicine was created to help bridge the gap and bring the two disciplines together. It may be a good choice for people who are looking for "the best of both worlds."

Several nations have attempted to synthesize traditional and modern medicine. Nations such as India and South Korea have successfully regulated traditional and complementary medicines into their national health policies.

- *Alternative Medicine:* This describes medical practices that replace conventional Western medicine. It refers to any form of medicine or healing that does not fall into conventional medical practice. An example is using a special diet to treat cancer instead of cancer drugs that are prescribed by an oncologist. Alternative medicine is often called complementary medicine, complementary and alternative medicine (CAM), or non-mainstream medicine. When adopted outside of its traditional culture, traditional medicine is often referred as complementary and alternative medicine (CAM). Alternative medicine includes relaxation technique, chiropractic, massage, spiritual healing, and weight-loss program as well as the use of herbs, vitamins, diets, hypnosis, energy, acupuncture, homeopathy, and folk remedies

- *Complementary Medicine:* This refers to practices outside Western medicine, adopted from other cultures. People seek complementary medicine for various ailments such as using herbal remedies to cure a cold or employing acupuncture to ease lower back pain.

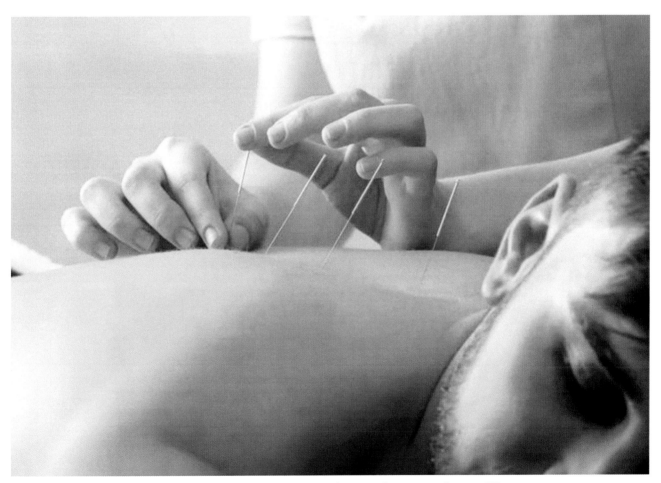

Figure 1.3 Acupuncture, a popular complementary therapy_[8].

Figure 1.3 illustrates acupuncture, a popular complementary therapy_[8]. Some people group "complementary and alternative medicine" (CAM) together. The use of CAM has continuously increased over the past decades. Many complementary therapies do not stand up to the standards of Western medicine. CAM includes therapies like acupuncture, yoga, meditation, massage, aromatherapy, traditional Chinese medicine, homeopathy, and chiropractic care. For example, traditional Chinese medicine (TCM) is indigenous to the Chinese. When TCM is used by non-Chinese, it becomes a complementary medicine. Some traditional and complementary medicines can negatively interact with other drugs. As shown in Figure 1.4, the reasons for preferring CAM to modern medicine include affordability, accessibility, acceptability, and effectiveness [9,10].

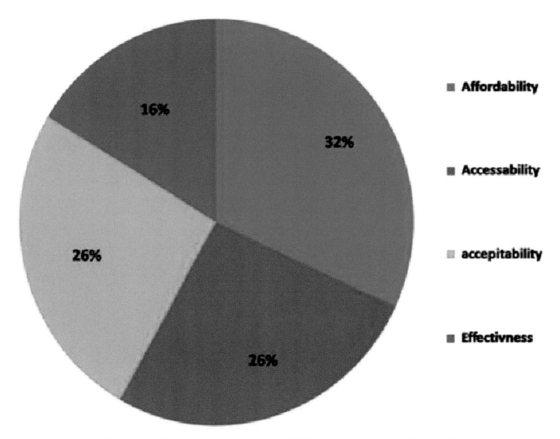

Figure 1.4 Reasons for preferring CAM to modern medicine [9].

- *Holistic Medicine:* "Holistic" denotes an approach that addresses the uniqueness of each individual and seeks to understand whole people in their total environments. Holistic medicine refers to treatment that considers a person's health as a whole, rather than focusing on one organ or bodily system. Some types of traditional, complementary, and integrative medicine are also holistic.

1.4 CONCEPT OF TRADITIONAL MEDICINES

Traditional medicine is a health practice with strong historical and cultural roots. It is the way of protecting and restoring health before the arrival of modern medicine. It refers to a range of practices and therapies indigenous to their practicing population. It has been used for centuries to ward off diseases and pathogens. It uses remedies derived from plants, animals, metals, and minerals. Traditional knowledge of indigenous medicine is handed down through ancestors, and was developed according to personal experiences. Traditional healers usually know their patients, their backgrounds, lifestyles, and cultural beliefs.

Traditional medicines have been classified into four categories [11]:

- *Category 1:* Traditional medicines that are prepared by a traditional health practitioner for an individual patient with fresh or dried raw materials, with a short shelf life.
- *Category 2:* Traditional medicines currently used in the community that are prepared in advance and composed of crude raw plant materials.
- *Category 3:* Standardized plant extracts prepared in advance and supported by scientific research.
- *Category 4:* Isolated pure compound molecules from traditional medicines following scientific research.

1.5 TRADITIONAL MEDICINES AROUND THE WORLD

Traditional systems of medicine are those that are unique or indigenous to a particular community or culture. Globally, various types of traditional medical practices exist. Some traditional medicines are supported by massive records of theoretical concepts and practical skills; others transmit orally from generation to generation through verbal teaching [11]. Examples of popular traditions medicines around the world are briefly discussed below [1,4, 12-15]:

- *Traditional Chinese Medicine:* TCM dates back to 200 B.C. China is regarded as one of the key players in advancing modern civilization, particularly in the area of scientific methodology. The country is endowed with a vast landscape with varied geographical features and a resultant wealth of medicinal plants. For example, in year 2010 alone, China manufactured 2.384 million tons of Chinese herbal products. Chinese medicine relies on the theory that the human body is an open organism operating in a continuous biological and mental exchange process with the outside environment. TCM differentiates signs and symptoms of a disease by 8 principles. It identifies different patterns of the evolution of disease by classifying factors of pathology according to climatic influences. Those factors are wind, cold, heat, dampness, dryness, and fire. For example, cold and heat, and Yin and Yang are two principles differentiating the nature of a disease, in that cold refers to syndromes caused by exogenous pathogenic cold, whereas heat represents syndromes caused by exogenous pathogenic heat. TCM prescribes formula for treating various diseases. TCM includes elements such as acupuncture, moxibustion, massage, relaxation, and herbal medicine. Today, the China Food and Drug Administration (CFDA) and the State Administration of Traditional Chinese Medicine (SATCM) regulate the TCM industry
- *Traditional Japanese Medicine:* TCM was brought to Japan through the Korean peninsula during the ancient era in the 5th century. Kampo medicine refers to Japanese traditional herbal medicine. It removed the speculative aspects of TCM and simplified the enormous amount of herbal medications available in TCM, reducing their complexity to about 300 extracts. By the middle of the 20th century, Kampo was simplified to a modern concept, which allowed understanding and acceptance for Western medicine trained doctors and physicians. Today, Kampo medicine courses are offered in all 80 medical schools from the Japanese universities.
- *Traditional Korean Medicine:* The traditional medicine in Korea evolves from two major philosophical traditions in China: Taoism and Confucianism. Taoism in medicine emphasizes nature, the universe, and therefore the environmental influences on health and disease. By contrast, Confucianism emphasizes the inner person, the strengths and weaknesses of the individual.

Korean traditional medicine is not very different from TCM in its use of herbal formulas and other treatments.

- *Traditional Indian Medicine:* Ayurveda is an Indian medical system with all regulatory procedures, related to health care, education, and quality standards of medicines in place. It consists of thousands of plants. Indians believe that "everything can be a drug." Many drugs such as levodopa, reserpine, chloroquin, aspirin, codeine, vincristin, vinblastin, bromohexine, and many others have their origins in Ayurveda, where they are used to treat the various diseases. The history of using plant resources for treating diseases in India can be dated back to 6,000 to 4,000 BCE, the Buddhist period. Advances made by medicine in India before the medieval era was truly substantial for surgery, healing knowledge, and tools. Today, Ayurveda is practiced across the country, particularly as the primary healthcare system for rural India.

- *Arabic Herbal Medicine:* The ancient Hippocratic-Greek medical knowhow was adapted and improved by Arabian herbalists in the Middle Ages. The Arabic world used to be the center of scientific and medical knowledge for many centuries (from 632 to 1258 CE). Arabs in the Baghdad region were the first in history to separate medicine from pharmacological science. The world's first drug stores were established in the Arab world. The practice of Arabic herbal medicine has been using natural remedies, both organic and inorganic types, for the prevention and treatment of diseases.

- *Traditional African Medicine:* Africa is home to diverse medicinal plants and herbs. These plant - or herb-based treatments have been a key part of the continent's traditional medicinal practices for thousands of years. Up to 80% of the people regularly use traditional medicines because they are accessible, affordable, and culturally accepted. Some people use traditional medicine in combination with Western medicines. Prescriptions of traditional African medicines tend to be secretive. They are based on knowledge passed orally from generation to generation of traditional healers, who implement herbs, spiritual healing, and minor surgical procedures in treating disease. The majority of healers rely on trade secrecy. An African traditional herbal medical practitioner is shown in Figure 1.5 [16]. Countries like Nigeria, Cameroon, Ethiopia, and South Africa have incorporated traditional African medicines into their healthcare systems. African Traditional Medicine day is celebrated every year in Cameroon and other places on the 31st August, to sensitize the public on the importance TM [17]. Burkina Faso, Cameroon, Democratic Congo, Guinea, Ghana, Madagascar, Mali, Nigeria, Rwanda, South Africa, and Togo have reported to be locally producing traditional medicines for the treatment of various diseases.

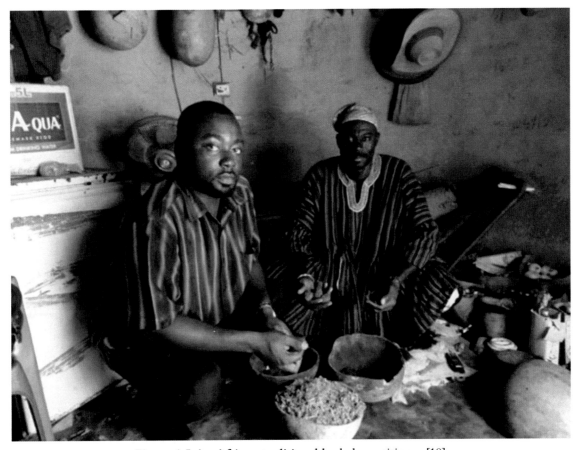

Figure 1.5 An African traditional herbal practitioner [10].

Other traditional medicines include Native American, South American, Mexican, Egyptian, Aboriginal, or Indonesian traditional medicines.

1.6 TRADITIONAL HERBS

Medicinal plants are the oldest known healthcare products. They have been an important contributor to the pharmaceutical, agricultural, and food industries. Herbalism is a traditional medicinal or folk medicine practice based on the use of plants and their extracts. It is the result of thousands of years of experience in practicing herbal medicine. Herbal medicine, also called botanical medicine, phytomedicine, refers to herbs and herbal products that contain plants and their extracts as active ingredients. The plant parts include seeds, berries, roots, stems, barks, heartwood, leaves, flower leaves, fruits, or even the whole plants. The physical properties of the herbal size, shape, color, texture, and taste traditionally helped in their selection for therapeutic purposes. The chemical ingredients residing in an herbal drug work with the body to maintain health or 5ht against diseases [1].

Numerous modern drugs originated from herbs or natural products. The herbal medicine is one element of complementary and alternative medicine. Many practitioners of traditional medicine have a deep knowledge of herbs and of their healing effects. The three major goals of using herbal medicine are to promote health, to prevent chronic or acute illness, and to treat them. Treating an illness is the most common goal for using herbal medicine. Figure 1.6 shows different forms and types of herbs used in tradition medicine [14].

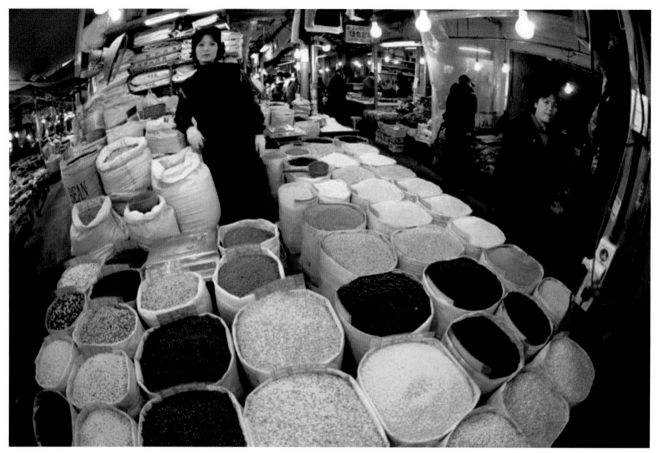

Figure 1.6 Different forms and types of herbs used in tradition medicine [12].

Some popular herbs are presented as follows [18-20]:

- *Echinacea* (or coneflower) is a flowering plant frequently used to treat and prevent cold. It has long been used in Native American practices to treat a variety of ailments, including wounds, burns, toothaches, and sore throat.
- *Ginseng* is a medicinal plant whose roots are frequently utilized in traditional Chinese medicine to boost immunity, brain function, and energy levels. It is also used to reduce inflammation.
- *Ginkgo biloba* is an herbal medicine derived from the maidenhair tree. It has been used in traditional Chinese medicine and remains a top-selling herbal supplement today because it treats a wide range of ailments, including heart disease, dementia, mental difficulties, memory loss, and sexual dysfunction. Figure 1.7 shows ginkgo biloba, a commonly used herb [18].

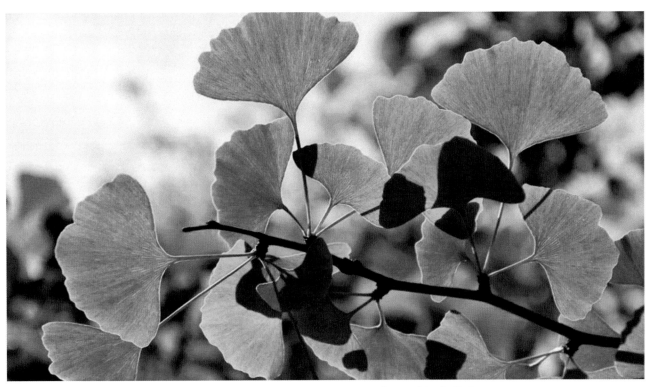

Figure 1.7 Ginkgo biloba, a commonly used herb [16].

- *Garlic* has been valued for centuries for its medicinal properties. It has demonstrated multiple beneficial cardiovascular effects. It has also been studied in hypertensive patients as a blood pressure–lowering agent. Besides garlic odor on the breath and body, moderate garlic consumption causes few adverse effects.
- *Elderberry* is an ancient herbal medicine used to treat cold and flu symptoms and relieve headaches, nerve pain, toothaches, colds, viral infections, and constipation.
- *Turmeric* is an herb that belongs to the ginger family. It is renowned for its anti-inflammatory benefits and may be effective for treating pain associated with arthritis.
- *Ginger* is a common ingredient and herbal medicine. It contains several active plant compounds and may treat a variety of conditions such as colds, nausea, migraines, and high blood pressure.
- *Valerian* is a flowering plant whose roots are thought to induce tranquility. Valerian root is often used as a natural sleep and anti-anxiety aid,
- *Chamomile* is a flowering plant and is one of the most popular herbal medicines in the world. It is used to treat a broad range of ailments.
- *Artemisinin* (Chinese sweet wormwood) is the basis for the most effective malaria drugs in the world. It is also proving useful against other diseases, including cancers and schistosomiasis
- *Hypericum perforatum* (known as St John's Wort) is a popular herbal supplement for treating depression in some cases. It is also used for anxiety and insomnia.
- *Reserpine* has been a Hindu Ayurvedic remedy since ancient times. It was one of the first drugs used on a large scale to treat systemic hypertension. It lowers blood pressure by decreasing cardiac output, peripheral vascular resistance, heart rate, and renin secretion.

Some of these herbs can eaten as fresh or dried. They may take the forms of a tea or capsule. Increasing demand for traditional medicine has important implications for the conservation of these herbs. Unfortunately, many plant species on earth have become endangered due to high consumption of herbs. Several herbal remedies have not undergone careful scientific evaluation and some cause serious toxic effects and major drug-to-drug interactions.

The following precautions must be taken in choosing herbal supplements [19]:

- Educate yourself and learn as much as you can about the herbs.
- Talk to your doctor before taking herbal supplements.
- Work with a professional and seek out the services of a trained and licensed herbalist.
- Consult with your pharmacist about the safety and effectiveness of the herbal medicine.
- Do not self-diagnose any health conditions.
- Watch for side effects. Be alert for allergic reactions.
- Purchase herbal medicine products from a reputable supplier.
- Be extra careful is buying herbal medicines over the Internet.
- Be cautious about buying herbal medicines or supplements manufactured overseas.
- Take all herbal medicines strictly as prescribed and consult your health practitioner immediately if you experience any side effects.
- Be aware of herbal medicine that can interact with other medications.

1.7 APPLICATIONS OF TRADITIONAL MEDICINE

Due to its pervasive nature, traditional medicine may have large public health impacts throughout the world. Communities around the world use traditional medicine for a variety of health problems, from warding off diseases to treating infectious diseases like pneumonia. TM is commonly used when modern medicine is ineffective, unavailable or unaffordable or when it provides effective and acceptable treatments for some conditions. The following are typical applications of TM [20,21]:

- In China, traditional Chinese medicine is used for the treatment of heart disease and stroke, chronic heart failure. arthritis, diabetes, hypertension, and cataracts. Traditional medicine is used as adjuvant therapy to modern medicine in China.
- India is the nation with the greatest reported use of TM. 11.7% of people reported that their most frequent source of care was TM.
- In Ghana, those of a lower socio-economic status, who are unemployed, live in rural areas, and report low health status, are more likely to use of traditional healers.
- Everyone is concerned these days about what COVID-19 is doing to society and how to fight against it. Different preparations from TCM have been evaluated for their use in treating COVID-19.
- In African countries like Zambia, Zimbabwe and South Africa, traditional medicine is widely used in the treatment of diseases such as HIV/AIDS and TB, especially as it is believed to generally improve quality of life in the patients.
- In European Union, various traditional herbal medicinal products exist in many member states. For these products, national authorities usually verify the safety and ensure a sufficient level of quality. For example, a specific simplified procedure exists in Austria, Belgium, France, and Germany.

- In United States, a product is primarily classified based on its intended use. For a botanical product, this intended use may be as a food (including a dietary supplement), a drug (including a biological drug), a medical device (e.g., gutta-percha) or a cosmetic. Most botanical products are marketed as dietary supplements.

- Nations in Africa, Asia and Latin America use traditional medicine to help meet some of their primary healthcare needs. TM is used in Africa when a disease cannot be treated by traditional medicine. For example, in Mexico the government is building regional health centers, which are staffed by traditional healers who are well trained.

- For cardiovascular diseases, herbal have been used in patients with congestive heart failure, systolic hypertension, cerebral insufficiency, venous insufficiency, and arrhythmia. However, cardiovascular disease is a serious health problem and no herbal remedy regimen should be initiated without careful consideration of its potential impact. Some herbs have adverse cardiovascular reactions and drug interactions.

- Obesity is a common global health problem, which is linked to cardiovascular and cerebrovascular diseases. It is a metabolic disorder characterized by an excess accumulation of fat in the body due to energy intake exceeding energy expenditure. Many studies have confirmed that herbal medicine is effective in the treatment of obesity.

1.8 BENEFITS

Traditional medicine has been used to treat cardiovascular diseases, anxiety, nervousness, insomnia, pain, respiratory disorders, sexually transmitted infections, tuberculosis, impotency, intestinal parasites, skin problems, liver diseases, mental disorders, hypertension, diabetes, and muscle tension. It has much to offer global health. It has been used in many nations throughout the world over many centuries. It makes significant contribution to the health promotion in present-day over-populated and aging societies. Global pharmaceutical companies have started to rediscover herbs as a potential source of new drug candidates. Other benefits include the following [22,23]:

- *Low Cost:* Although the use of modern medicine has increased, it is not easily accessible for much of the population due to prohibitively high costs and limited availability, especially in rural areas. Traditional medicines provide affordable means of primary healthcare to poor and marginalized people in impoverished rural areas.

- *Harmless Treatment:* Traditional medicines are harmless. They have been used for the treatment of many common and complex diseases with a minimum of adverse side effects compared to conventional drugs. They are used for treating mild to moderate diseases for all ages and to prevent illness and promote health for the elderly.

- *Simple Treatment:* Herbal medicine is so simple that it appears to be self-medicated treatment for which a user can become an expert by consulting books, family members, or Internet. Traditional herbs are often packaged in the form of powders, capsules, salves, and tonics to be self-administered. Today, many practitioners of conventional medicine do not hesitate to recommend herbs and herbal products

- *Decentralized Treatment:* Traditional medicine is decentralized. It is readily available to individuals for whom traveling to urban centers for treatment is inconvenient, time-consuming, and costly.

- *Dual Medical Systems*: Due to the benefits of traditional medicine, many countries have allowed a dual system of medical care in which individuals can choose between traditional or Western clinics.

1.9 CHALLENGES

The drawbacks of traditional medicine include incorrect diagnosis, improper dosage, low hygiene standards, and the secrecy of some healing methods [14]. A common criticism of traditional medicine is that medical doctors treat symptoms instead of looking for the root cause of the symptoms. The current challenge is to pursue action along three lines: evaluation, integration, and training. Efforts should be made integrate traditional and modern medicines. Traditional practitioners also require training.

The globalization of traditional medicine affects both the quality control of medicaments and the training and competence of practitioners. There are challenges in coding and classifying traditional and herbal medicines. Another major problem for both physicians and patients has been the paucity of scientific data on herbal medicines used in the United States. Excessive medical treatment and medication, including the consumption of herbal medications, is a global trend, especially in developed countries.

Other challenges include the following [24]:

- *Safety:* This is the likelihood of a traditional medicine not causing harm. The increasing use and popularity of traditional medicine have created challenges in public health from the point of view of politics, safety, efficacy, quality, access, and rational use. Safety of some herbal medicines has been recently called into question.
- *Scientific Validation:* This is necessary for useful interpretation and wider acceptance of TM. Evidence is the major component in evidence-based medicine and practice. The acceptance of traditional medicine by the scientific community is limited by the lack of ground-breaking scientific validation of its efficacy. The quality and efficacy data on traditional medicine are far from sufficient to meet the criteria needed to support its use worldwide. Analytical methods should be developed to evaluate the safety and efficacy of various elements of traditional medicine.
- *Standardization:* Modern medicine demands standard dosages. Herbal medicine has been challenged by practitioners of mainstream medicine because of the lack of scientific evidence. Considerable benefits are possible when the local medicinal plants are subjected to scientific methods of validation and standardization of traditional use and quality control.
- *Ethics:* The ethical principles governing traditional medicine research demand that researchers must respect, preserve, and maintain traditional knowledge, innovations, and practices.
- *Culture Clash:* Traditional medicine is often regarded as clinically ineffective by modern standards. Scientific research on traditional medicines does not always fit the Western model for medical research. Health insurance coverage is very difficult to justify if traditional medicine products and practices are not evidence-based.
- *Regulation:* Universal regulation is nearly impossible. Efforts to make traditional medicines mainstream need to cope with varying regulation as each nation follows different rules. Methods for evaluating and regulating medicines vary widely. What is traditional for one group may not

be traditional for another in the same nation. Governments should establish systems for qualifying and licensing of traditional medicine practitioners.

* *Overexploitation:* The practice of herbal medicine involves using more than 53,000 species. Unfortunately, a great number of these species on earth are facing the threat of extinction due to overexploitation.

Figure 1.8 illustrates some of these challenges.

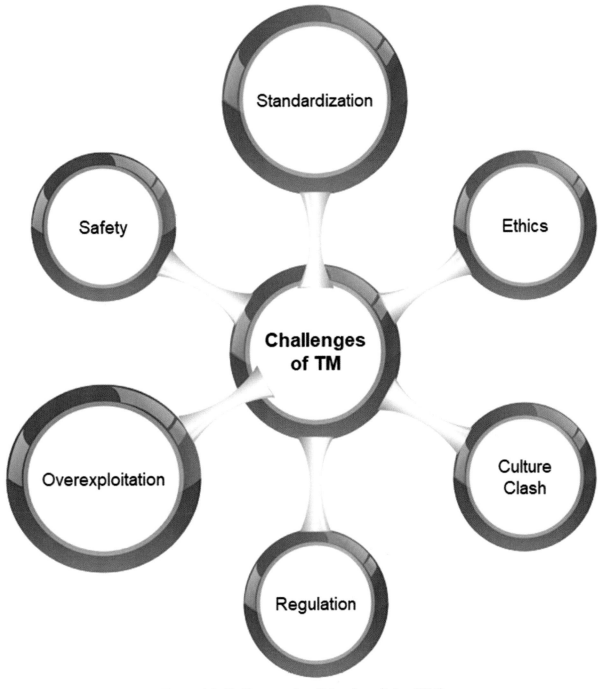

Figure 1.8 Challenges of traditional medicine (TM).

1.10 GLOBAL NEED OF TRADITIONAL MEDICINE

The use of traditional medicines has expanded globally. Practices of traditional medicine vary greatly from nation to nation, as they are influenced by factors such as culture, history, personal attitudes, and philosophy. Traditional medicine occupies a very important place in healthcare in the world in general, in developing nations in particular. It is an indispensable healthcare component in low-income countries. In view of the benefits of traditional medicine, many nations in Asia, Africa, and South America have developed a dual healthcare system in which patients can choose whether they visit traditional or Western clinics.

Traditional medical knowledge is attracting attention worldwide due to global healthcare demand and the significant role of TM in meeting the public health needs of developing countries. Traditional Knowledge Digital Library (TKDL) is first of its kind to make the knowledge available in English and other languages. Traditional medicine has much to offer global health. WHO has been increasingly involved in developing international standards and technical guidelines for traditional medicines in order to implement the slogan "Health for all by the year AD 2000" [9]. In 1992, the WHO invited a group of experts to develop criteria and general principles to guide research work on evaluating herbal medicines.

Education and research on traditional medicine have advanced. About 40 nations now provide high-level education and training programs on traditional medicine. Some medical schools offer some courses on various aspects of traditional and complementary medicine at undergraduate and graduate levels. They are serious about integrating traditional medicine into modern healthcare [14].

1.11 ORGNIZATIONS SUPPORTING TM

The use of herbal medicine, as one element of complementary and alternative medicine, is increasing worldwide. Several traditional medicine institutions and organizations are involved in the process of developing and advancing TM. Each national government should take steps to regulate and control TM products with a view to ensuring their safety, efficacy, and quality. It should establish the necessary institutional and financial support to promote traditional medicine in its healthcare delivery. The government may develop guidelines on regulating herbal medicines, in consultation with traditional healers and researchers. For example, the Department for Traditional Medicine within the National Institute for Research on Public Health was created in Mali. In 1847, the American Medical Association (AMA) was created to try to regulate medical care. The AMA urges doctors and the public to be well informed about the therapies they use to treat illnesses. The FDA considers herbal supplements foods, not drugs. We only consider the following international bodies that promote TM [25]:

- *World Health Organization* (WHO): WHO is well aware that many elements of traditional medicine are beneficial while others are not. In this respect, the Organization encourages and supports countries in their efforts to find safe and effective remedies for their healthcare services. WHO Traditional Medicine Strategy 2014–2023 provides the following set of definitions [26]:
  - ➢ *Traditional and complementary medicine:*
  - ➢ Traditional and complementary medicine include herbs, herbal materials, herbal preparations, and finished herbal products that contain parts of plants, other plant materials, or combinations thereof as active ingredients.

➤ *Traditional medicine:*
➤ Traditional medicine has a long history. It is the sum total of the knowledge, skill, and practices based on the theories, beliefs, and experiences indigenous to different cultures, whether explicable or not, used in the maintenance of health as well as in the prevention, diagnosis, improvement, or treatment of physical and mental illness.
➤ *Complementary medicine*

The terms "complementary medicine" or "alternative medicine" refer to a broad set of healthcare practices that are not part of that country's own tradition or conventional medicine and are not fully integrated into the dominant healthcare system. They are used interchangeably with traditional medicine in some countries.

Since 1975, WHO has emphasized the importance of maintaining traditional medicines in the healthcare systems of underdeveloped countries. In 1978, WHO along with UNICEF urged its member states to foster collaboration between traditional and western systems of care. It emphasized five major areas of concern: national program development; health systems and operational research; clinical and scientific investigations; education and training; and exchange of information. Since the 1970s, WHO has supported training in acupuncture by establishing collaborating centers. In order to ensure the safe and effective use of traditional medicine, WHO supports research and training activities. A WHO global survey report on Traditional Medicine/Complementary and Alternative Medicine (TM/CAM) of 2005 raised valuable concerns on the issue of safety, drug efficacy, and quality control.

• *International Regulatory Cooperation for Herbal Medicines*: In 2006, WHO established a this global network to allow communication and exchange between worldwide regulatory authorities responsible for the regulation of herbal medicines.
• *European Cooperation in the Field of Scientific and Technical research* (COST): This was set up by the European Commission to improve pan-European collaboration in science and technology. The COST group was established in June 1993 with a mandate to investigate the therapeutic significance of unconventional medicine, its cost-benefit ratio, and its sociocultural importance.

1.12 CONCLUSION

Traditional medicine is a major foundation on which modern medicine has been built. The use of traditional medicine for health purposes has increased in both developing and developed countries. Herbs as a resource remain the indispensable resource from which even alternative medicines are derive. Herbal products are widely available to consumers and have become increasingly popular throughout the world. It is due for a revival. If both developed and developing nations collaborate on traditional medicine research and development, new scientific techniques could spark a revival in global healthcare. More information about traditional medicine can be found in the books in [27-32] and the following related journals:

• *Journal of Herbal Medicine*
• *Journal of Ethnopharmacology.*
• *Journal of Alternative and Complementary Medicine*

- *Chinese Journal of Integrative Medicine*
- *African Journal of Traditional, Complementary and Alternative Medicines*
- *Advances in Traditional Medicine*
- *Traditional Medicine and Modern Medicine*

REFERENCES

[1] S. Y. Pan et al., "Historical perspective of traditional indigenous medical practices: The current renaissance and conservation of herbal resources," *Evidence-Based Complementary and Alternative Medicine*, vol. 2014, 2014.

[3] M. N. O. Sadiku, O. D. Olaleye, A. Ajayi-Majebi, and S. M. Musa, "Traditional Medicine: A Primer," *International Journal of Trend in Research and Development,* vol. 8, no. 5, November–December 2021, pp. 341-346.

[4] N. Lemonnier, "Traditional knowledge-based medicine: A review of history, principles, and relevance in the present context of P4 systems medicine," *Progress in Preventive Medicine,* vol 2, no. 7, December 2017.

[5] M. Leonti and R. Verpoorte, "Traditional Mediterranean and European herbal medicines," *Journal of Ethnopharmacology,* vol. 199, March 2017, pp. 161-167.

[6] "Complementary and alternative medicine,"
https://www.cancer.gov/about-cancer/treatment/cam

[7] "Alternative vs. Traditional medicine,"
https://www.winchesterhospital.org/health-library/article?id=13500

[8] J. Agu, "Traditional medicines must be integrated into health care for culturally diverse groups," May 2019,
https://theconversation.com/traditional-medicines-must-be-integrated-into-health-care-for-culturally-diverse-groups-114980

[9] N. Belachew, T. Tadesse, and A. A. Gube, "Knowledge, attitude, and practice of complementary and alternative medicine among residents of Wayu town, Western Ethiopia," *Journal of Evidence-Based Complementary and Alternative Medicine,* vol. 22, no. 4, October 2017, pp.929–935.

[10] C. T. Che et al., "Traditional medicine," *Pharmacognosy,* 2017.

[11] T. Che et al., " Chapter 2 - Traditional medicine," *Pharmacognosy,* 2017, pp. 15-30.

[12] "Traditional medicine for modern times: Facts and figures," June 2015,
https://www.scidev.net/global/features/traditional-medicine-modern-times-facts-figures/

[13] C. Gouws, "Traditional African medicine and conventional drugs: Friends or enemies?" March 2018,
https://theconversation.com/traditional-african-medicine-and-conventional-drugs-friends-or-enemies-92695

[14] G. O. Essegbey, "The dynamics of innovation in traditional medicine in Ghana," February 2015,
https://www.wipo.int/wipo_magazine/en/2015/01/article_0003.html

[15] C. N. Fokunang, "Traditional medicine: Past, present and future research and development prospects and integration in the national health system of Cameroon," *African Journal of Traditional, Complementary and Alternative Medicines, v*ol. 8, no. 3, 2011, pp. 284–295.

[16] A. Hill, "9 of the world's most popular herbal medicines," February 2020, https://www.healthline.com/nutrition/herbal-medicine

[17] "Herbal medicine," https://www.betterhealth.vic.gov.au/health/conditionsandtreatments/herbal-medicine

[18] Ni. H. Mashour, G. I. Lin, and W. H. Frishman, "Herbal medicine for the treatment of cardiovascular disease: Clinical considerations," *Archives of Internal Medicine,* vol. 158, no. 20, November 1998, pp. 2225-2234.

[19] "Herbal medicine," https://www.hopkinsmedicine.org/health/wellness-and-prevention/herbal-medicine

[20] O. Oyebode et al., "Use of traditional medicine in middle-income countries: A WHO-SAGE study," *Health Policy and Planning,* vol. 31, no. 8, October 2016, pp. 984–991.

[21] Y. Liu et al., "Herbal medicine for the treatment of obesity: An overview of scientific evidence from 2007 to 2017," *Evidence-Based Complementary and Alternative Medicine,* vol. 2017, 2017.

[22] D. Young. I. Grant, and S. Ingelise, "The persistence of traditional medicine in the modern world," *Cultural Survival Quarterly Magazine* March 1988, https://www.culturalsurvival.org/publications/cultural-survival-quarterly/persistence-traditional-medicine-modern-world

[23] A. N. Welz, A. Emberger-Klein, and K. Menrad, "Why people use herbal medicine: Insights from a focus-group study in Germany," *BMC Complementary and Alternative Medicine,* vol. 18, 2018.

[24] O. Akerele, " WHO's traditional medicine programme: Progress and perspectives," *WHO Chronicle,* vol. 38, no. 2, 1984, pp. 76-81.

[25] X. Zhang, "Traditional medicine and WHO," *World Health,* no. 2, March-April, 1996.

[26] W. Knoess and J. Wiesner, "The globalization of traditional medicines: Perspectives related to the European union regulatory environment," *Engineering,* vol.5, no. 1, 2019, pp. 22-31.

[27] K. B. Barimah and O. Bonna, *Traditional Medicine in Ghana.* CreateSpace Independent Publishing Platform, 2018.

[28] R. C. Croizier, *Traditional Medicine in Modern China: Science, Nationalism, and the Tensions of Cultural Change.* Cambridge, MA: Harvard University Press, 2013.

[29] A. Chevallier, *Encyclopedia of Herbal Medicine: 550 Herbs and Remedies for Common Ailments.* DK; 3rd edition, 2016.

[30] J. Qiu, *Traditional Medicine: A Culture in the Balance.* Nature Publishing Group, 2007.

[31] J. A. Duke, *Handbook of Medical Herbs.* Boca Raton, FL: CRC Press, 2002.

[32] A. Garlow, *The Native American Herbalist's Bible: 5 in 1 - The Only Guide You Need to Live an Healthy Life by Discovering the Native Americans Remedies, Best Herbal Recipes & Essential Oils.* Independently Published, 2021.

2
CHAPTER

Traditional Chinese Medicine

"If current Chinese medicine became the standard under international agreement, it would have an impact on our education and qualification & systems." Katsutoshi Terasawa,

2.1 INTRODUCTION

The need for culturally competent healthcare is vital. Traditional Chinese medicine (TCM) is perhaps the most popular and well-research traditional medicine. It is one of the acknowledged natural medicines classified by World Health Organization (WHO). It is a comprehensive medical practices which have been developed in China for more than 2,000 years to prevent, diagnose, and treat disease. This healthcare system is becoming popular in recent years throughout Asia, Europe, India, Africa, and the Americas. It is more accessible, more affordable, and more acceptable to people. It has great potential to improve health and wellness. TCM is fully integrated into the healthcare systems of China, South Korea, North Korea, and Japan [1,2].

Traditional Chinese medicine (TCM) originated from traditional Chinese culture and has evolved over thousands of years. It is a rich medical system that includes various forms of herbal medicine, acupuncture, massage, exercise, and dietary therapy. This heritage has been incorporated into modern development and practices of medicine. TCM is designed for restoring the balance of the body for sick people and maintain health for others. Some of its precepts were standardized in the People's Republic of China, where the government promoted a systematized form of TCM. TCM has influenced traditional systems of medicine in other Asian countries such as Japan and Korea. In the United States, people use TCM essentially as a complementary health approach or as dietary supplements. In contrast to modern Western medicine, Chinese traditional medicine is designed to restore the balance of human body n order to achieve the state of health. Figure 2.1 shows a comparison between TCM and modern western medicine.

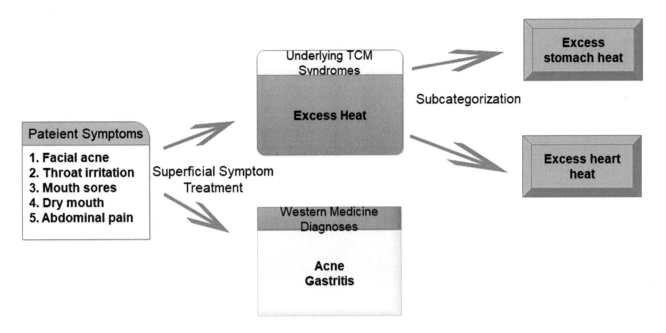

Figure 2.1 A comparison between TCM and modern western medicine.

This chapter provides a brief introduction to traditional Chinese medicine. It begins by providing a brief history and underlying concepts of Chinese medicine. It covers the eight principles of diagnosis. It discusses herbal medicine. It provides some applications of TCM. It presents the modernization of TCM. It highlights its benefits and challenges. It concludes with comments.

2.2 BRIEF HISTORY OF TCM

TCM in an ancient medical practice. The origin of Chinese medical practice was closely related to Chinese ancestors in the primitive era. Over the years, the traditional Chinese medicine (TCM) has evolved into a complex medical system with its own understanding of anatomy, physiology, pathology and therapeutics. TCM is widely used in Greater China, where it has a long history. The first, and perhaps one of the most important, textbook of TCM was completed in about 200 BC. This treatise, known as the Yellow Emperor's Classic of Internal Medicine (Huang Di Nei Jing Tai Su), provides the reader with theory and philosophy of TCM. The first, and perhaps one of the most important, textbook of TCM was completed in about 200 BC. This treatise, known as the Yellow Emperor's Classic of Internal Medicine provides the reader with theory and philosophy of TCM [4].

In the 19th century, Chinese people migrated to the United States to work. With them came Chinese medicine, which was then practiced exclusively in Chinese communities. Chinese medicine remained relatively unknown to the American public until the early 1970's. Many Americans only became aware of TCM through the practice of acupuncture during the 1970s.

In the 1950s, the Chinese government promoted a systematized form of TCM. In 1950, Chairman Mao Zedong declared his support for traditional Chinese medicine (TCM) even though he did not personally believe in TCM and he did not use it. In the 1950's and 60's, the Chinese government codified traditional Chinese medicine.

In 2006, the Chinese scholar Zhang Gongyao triggered a national debate when he published an article entitled "Farewell to Traditional Chinese Medicine," arguing that TCM should be abolished in public healthcare. The Chinese government took the position that TCM is a science and continued to encourage its development. As of 2007 there were not enough good-quality trials of herbal therapies to allow their effectiveness to be determined. Today, China is at a critical stage of reforming its medical system.

2.3 UNDERLYING CONCEPTS

TCM arose from the naturalistic philosophies of ancient China and is based on the following abstract concepts. The most important concepts taken from ancient Chinese naturalistic philosophy in TCM are those of qi, yinyang, and the five phases (wuxing). The upper body is yang in relation to the lower body, which is yin. The human body is a miniature version of the larger, surrounding universe. Human beings are part of nature. The body has its own alarms or reactions to malfunctions. TCM is based on the concept that the human body consists of interconnected systems which maintain healthy function through the balance of yin and yang, or opposing energies. When yin and yang are out of balance, health is adversely affected. Disease is regarded as a deviation from natural conditions. Sound health is understood as the proper balance of contending forces. Life arises from the polar forces Yang and Yin, Heaven and Earth, heat and cold, sun and shadow, dryness and wetness, summer and winter [4].

Five elements or five phases —fire, earth, wood, metal, and water—symbolically represent all phenomena including the stages of human life. These are illustrated in Figure 2.2.

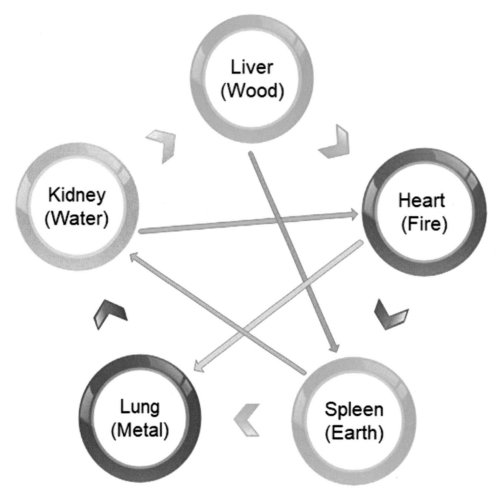

Figure 2.2 Basic principles or elements of TCM .

Figure 2.3 shows the display table in the Kampo Museum shows the relationship between the Five Chinese elements, the different parts of the body they are related to and the herbs that can be used to treat a range of ailments [6]. The six excesses and their characteristic clinical signs are [7]:

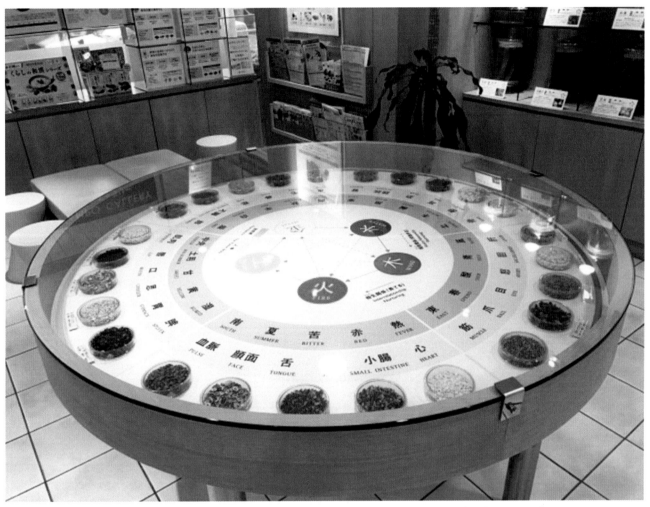

Figure 2.3 The display table in the Kampo Museum shows the relationship between the Five Chinese elements, e related to and the herbs that can be used to treat a range of ailments [6].

1. *Wind:* Rapid onset of symptoms, wandering location of symptoms, itching, nasal congestion; tremor, paralysis, convulsion.
2. *Cold*: Cold sensations, aversion to cold, relief of symptoms by warmth, watery/clear excreta, severe pain, and abdominal pain. Cold is usually characterized by aversion to cold, absence of thirst.
3. *Fire/Heat*: Aversion to heat, high fever, thirst, concentrated urine, red face, red tongue, yellow tongue fur, rapid pulse.
4. *Dampness*: Sensation of heaviness, sensation of fullness, greasy tongue fur, "slippery" pulse.
5. *Dryness*: Dry cough, dry mouth, dry throat, dry lips, nosebleeds, dry skin, dry stools.
6. *Summerheat*: Either heat or mixed damp–heat symptoms.

Six-Excesses can also transform from one into another. Extreme wind, heat, and cold can wreak havoc and derange balance within the human body.

The four key TCM principles are [8]: (1) Your body is an integrated whole, (2) You are completely connected to nature, (3) You were born with a natural self-healing ability, (4) Prevention is the best cure.

TCM practitioners use various techniques to promote health and treat disease. These include diet, herbal medicine, acupuncture, acupressure, moxibustion, meditation, physical exercise, and massage. In the United States, the most commonly used approaches include Chinese herbal medicine, acupuncture, and tai chi [9].

- *Herbal medicine:* Herbal treatment is basic to TCM treatment. It consists of plants, minerals, and animal products. This also includes some human parts. The substances can come from different leaves, roots, stems, flowers, and seeds of plants.
- *Acupuncture:* This is another cornerstone in TCM. It is a family of procedures involving the stimulation of specific points on the body using a variety of techniques. Acupuncture involves inserting fine thin needles into superficial structures (skin, tissue, and muscles) of the body and their subsequent manipulation. In electroacupuncture, an electric current is applied to the needles to further stimulate.
- *Tai chi:* This is a centuries-old mind and body practice. It involves gentle, dance-like body movements with mental focus, breathing, and relaxation. Tai chi has not been investigated as extensively as acupuncture or Chinese herbal medicine. TCM has been fully integrated into the health care systems of China, South Korea, North Korea, and Japan. The practice of TCM is regulated in most states in the US. License is granted to the practitioners whose practices are recognized as safe and bring the benefit for health.

2.4 EIGHT PRINCIPLES OF DIAGNOSIS

Diagnosis aims at determining the prevailing balance within the ecosystem of an individual by assessing the quantity and quality of Qi . In TCM, Zheng is a distinct diagnostic concept. Zheng is more specific than the eight principles. The first and most important step in pattern diagnosis is an evaluation of the present signs and symptoms on the basis of the "Eight Principles." Every principle reflects and harmonizes with the relationships that exist within natural law. The TCM practitioners use these principles of diagnosis in their assessments, including looking, listening, smelling, asking, and touching. The eight principles refer to four pairs of fundamental qualities of a disease: exterior/interior, heat/cold, vacuity/repletion, and yin/yang. The Eight Principles refer to the following [4]:

- *Yin and yang* are universal aspects all things can be classified under, this includes diseases in general as well as the Eight Principles' first three couples. For example, cold is identified to be a yin aspect, while heat is attributed to yang.
- *Exterior* refers to a disease manifesting in the superficial layers of the body – skin, hair, flesh, and meridians. It is characterized by aversion to cold and/or wind, headache, muscle ache, mild fever, and a normal tongue appearance.
- *Interior* refers to disease manifestation in the zàng-fŭ to any disease that cannot be counted as exterior.
- *Cold* is generally characterized by aversion to cold, absence of thirst, and a white tongue fur.
- *Heat* is characterized by absence of aversion to cold, a red and painful throat, a dry tongue fur and a rapid and floating pulse.

- *Deficiency* an be further differentiated into deficiency of qi, xuě, yin, and yang, with all their respective characteristic symptoms.
- *Excess* generally refers to any disease that cannot be identified as a deficient pattern. In a concurrent exterior pattern, excess is characterized by the absence of sweating.

After the fundamental nature of a disease in terms of the Eight Principles is determined, the investigation focuses on more specific aspects.

2.5 HERBAL MEDICINE

Chinese herbal medicine (CHM) plays an important role of treatment in traditional Chinese medicine (TCM). Traditionally, CHM is used to restore the balance of the body for sick people and maintain health for common people. Chinese herbs primarily come from different parts of the plants, including leaves, roots, stems, flowers, and seeds. The source or origin and quality of the traditional herbs have a direct impact on the efficacy of TCM.

The term "herbal medicine" is somewhat misleading in that, while plant elements are by far the most commonly used substances in TCM, other, non-botanic substances are used as well: animal, human, and mineral products. There are roughly 13,000 medicinals used in China and over 100,000 medicinal recipes recorded in the ancient literature. Plant elements and extracts are by far the most common elements used. Some medicines can include the parts of endangered species, including tiger bones. The illegal trade for tiger parts in China has driven the species to near-extinction because of its popularity in TCM. TCM also includes some human parts such as bones, fingernail, hairs, dandruff, earwax, impurities on the teeth, feces, urine, sweat, and organs.

The top 10 kinds of most frequently used herbs included [10]: (1) Radix Glycyrrhizae (Gancao), (2) Poria (Fuling), (3) Rhizoma Corydalis (Yanhusuo), (4) Radix Angelicae Sinensis (Danggui), (5) Radix Ginseng (Renshen), (6) Radix Astragali (Huangqi), (7) Rhizoma Atractylodis Macrocephalae (Baizhu), (8) Semen Ziziphi Spinosae (Suanzaoren), (9) Radix Polygalae (Yuanzhi) and (10) Flos Daturae (Yangjinhua).

Examples of commonly used herbs are shown in Figure 2.4[10].

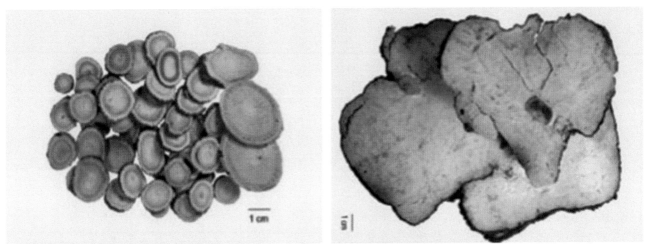

1. *Radix Glycyrrhizae (Gancao)*   2. *Poria (Fuling)*

Figure 2.4 Examples of commonly used herbs [10].

2.6 APPLICATIONS

Traditional Chinese medicine (TCM) is a complete system of healing that was developed in China about 2,000 years. It is getting more and more popular worldwide for improving health condition of human beings as well as preventing and healing diseases. Its use in diagnosis and treatment of diseases is fascinating because it emphasizes the harmony in human bodies. Traditional Chinese medicine believes that the status of one's health signifies the balance of Yin-Yang, while a condition of pathological state implies imbalance of Yin-Yang. Chinese medicine emphasizes the underlying connection of the bodily, emotional, social, and environmental dimensions in disease and healing. The following are common uses of TCM.

- *Acupuncture:* Acupuncture is the cornerstone of TCM diagnostic and treatment. It is a special branch of TCM, which has been extensively studied by practitioners. It is the practice of introducing thin needles into specific points of the body where the energy flows. In China today, TCM accounts for around 40% of all health care delivered and acupuncture is practiced side by side with Western medicine in hospitals and clinics. In the US, Chinese medicine is also becoming increasingly integrated with medical practices and used in conjunction with medical treatments. Chinese medical providers, commonly referred to as acupuncturists, are licensed in forty-four states in US and the District of Columbia. Sometimes acupuncture and herbs are used in tandem with prescription drugs; sometimes they can replace them. US-trained acupuncturists have provided emergency support in areas as diverse as Haiti, the US gulf coast, and Nepal. Acupuncture is being widely used in the medical community as a potential alternative or complementary treatment for many diseases. Acupuncture and herbal medicine are known to be helpful in health problems such as developmental retardation in children resulting from birth injury, meningitis, pain, infertility, colitis, stroke, flu, despair, irritability, and the side effects of chemotherapy and radiation. There are numerous challenges to achieving a consensus over the use of acupuncture in a medical environment. Additionally, a unified scientific theory to explain the diverse effects of acupuncture (from pain control to immunomodulation) is lacking [11]. An example of acupuncture is shown in Figure 2.5 [12].

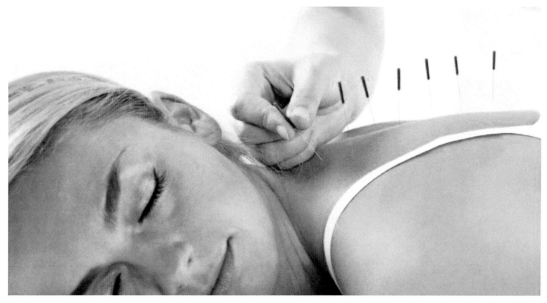

Figure 2.5 An example of acupuncture [12].

- *Tongue Diagnosis;* A TCM practitioner's analysis of the tongue will include its size, shape, tension, color, and coating. Below is a diagram of all the channels/meridians reaching the tongue areas that correspond to internal organs in TCM. The tongue has various features that indicate various bodily functions [13]:
  - ➤ Tongue body color: indicates the state of blood, organs, and Qi
  - ➤ Tongue body shape: reflects the state of blood and Qi, and indicates excess or deficiency
  - ➤ Tongue body features: teeth marks may indicate that the tongue rests against the teeth. This is often a sign of a digestive disorder or (e.g. red dots) may indicate heat or inflammation in the blood
  - ➤ Tongue body moisture: reveals the state of fluids in the body
  - ➤ Tongue coating: indicates the state of organs, especially the stomach
  - ➤ Tongue coat thickness (e.g. thick) may indicate an imbalance in digestion or (e.g. peeled) may be associated with allergic disorders and autoimmune diseases
  - ➤ Tongue body cracks: could be a sign of a yeast infection or a biotin deficiency
  - ➤ Tongue coat root: indicates impairment of organs if it is not attached to the tongue's surface

A typical example of tongue diagnose is depicted in Figure 2.6 [5].

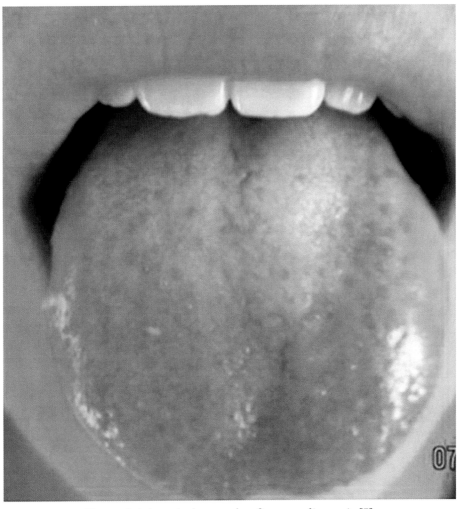

Figure 2.6 A typical example of tongue diagnosis [5].

- *Cancer:* There is no consensus on the exact causes of malignant tumors. Factors such as viruses, infections, heredity, psychology, diet, and the environment may be involved. Surgery, chemotherapy and radiotherapy are three major modern treatments of malignant tumors. Their primary aim is to destroy the tumor. TCM can play an important role in cancer prevention and treatment. It has been increasingly used in the last decades as a therapy to alleviate cancer symptoms at the terminal stages when Western medicine treatments cannot offer any other treatment options [14].
- *Alzheimer's disease* (AD): Alzheimer's disease (AD) is well known as a severe threat to the elderly. As the process of aging population and society, AD has become a serious threat to public health. Some kinds of Chinese herbal medicine might be potentially useful in treating Alzheimer's disease (AD) [15].
- *Pharmacology:* The traditional Chinese pharmacopoeia describes a large number of herbal formulations that are used for the treatment of various diseases. Most Chinese formulations contain a combination of the various herbs in defined proportions. Pharmaceutical companies have explored the potential for creating new drugs from TCM. TCM herbal product manufacturers provide products of reputable quality to the market. Different areas of classical pharmacy focus on medicinal herbs, e.g. phytochemistry, pharmacognosy and phytotherapy. Many secondary metabolites of plants exert pharmacological features. The exploitation of these beneficial effects is the goal of pharmacology of natural products. Natural products are among the major players in pharmacology [16]. The role of the drug in TCM is merely to either improve the body's regulatory mechanisms or remove factors that impair the self-healing ability of the body. The ultimate requirements of drugs should be efficacy and safety.

Other applications of the traditional Chinese medicine include dermatologic disorders, psychiatric disorders, anti-influenza, drug addiction, tuberculosis, and rheumatoid arthritis.

2.7 MODERNIZATION

Traditional Chinese medicine is medical system that has been practiced for centuries to prevent, diagnose, and treat disease. It should be regarded as an alternative method of therapy which can be administered in oral, topical, or injectable forms. It has been used to treat various conditions including malaria symptoms, jaundice, rheumatism, diabetic wounds, drug addiction, cancer, tuberculosis, and menstrual complications.

TCM has provided an new alternative way of looking at medical practices, health care, scientific research, education, industry, and culture. It has been continuously refined through observation, testing, and critical thinking. The Chinese government has undertaken efforts to modernize TCM. The health services of TCM are continuously developing and are becoming globalized at an accelerated pace [17]. It has faced the crisis and challenge of historical continuity and modernization. Since the end of 20th century China has started to collect medical data of TCM through computer.

Although TCM can be practiced as a stand-alone therapy, it functions best in close integration with Western medical care. In China, acupuncture is practiced side by side with Western medicine in hospitals and clinics. Recently, the Chinese government has made concerted efforts to modernize TCM by investing capital in scientific research and development of TCM. Interest in TCM is growing rapidly beyond China.

2.8 BENEFITS

TCM has many beneficial effects. It has been used for centuries and has been proved to be better efficacy and fewer adverse effects. It is known to treat the cause of a disease rather than to alleviate its symptoms. Traditional medical doctors usually apply a holistic approach in treating a patient. This medical approach is appropriate to disease prevention and the treatment of chronic diseases without collateral damage. TCM can be integrated with modern medical treatments of surgery, radiotherapy, chemotherapy, and molecular targeted therapy. Other benefits of TCM include the following [18]:

- *Philosophy:* TCM has its unique way of thinking. Unlike Western medicine, TCM is more of a philosophy than science. The human being is a microcosm and the offspring of Heaven and Earth. People are recognized as beings with a self-aware mind cast in physical form. Disease is understood to be a deviation from natural conditions. TCM provides a framework for understanding, interpreting, and organizing interventions in the human health-disease process.
- *Simplicity:* TCMs can be effectively applied to help heal anyone and any health issue. They are safe, simple, natural, nontoxic, and inexpensive. They can be taken for general well-being, not necessarily when one is sick.
- *Alternative Medicines:* Traditional Chinese medicines provides a distinct way to view our human life, disease, and treatment. They have played a significant role as alternative medicines.
- *Dissatisfaction with Western Medicine (WM):* Lack of satisfaction with the Western medicine (WM) is the most common reason for interest in alternative therapy. There is mounting evidence that supports that TCM is efficacious,
- *Broad Treatment:* TCM is not limited to pain management. World Health Organization (WHO) has listed problems such as bronchitis, flu, arthritis, stroke, infertility, dizziness, insomnia, and depression as amenable to acupuncture therapy.
- *Worldwide Acceptance:* There is a growing and sustained interest in TCM around the world. This interest is driven partly by dissatisfaction with the traditional Western medical model. TCMs are widely used around the world. The global role of TCM in primary healthcare has been recognized by the WHO. Several national governments (such as Canada, Australia Singapore, and Malaysia) have embraced, supported, and regulated TCM practice. They have integrated TCM into their healthcare system, while also using conventional Western medical therapies.

These benefits are illustrated in Figure 2.7.

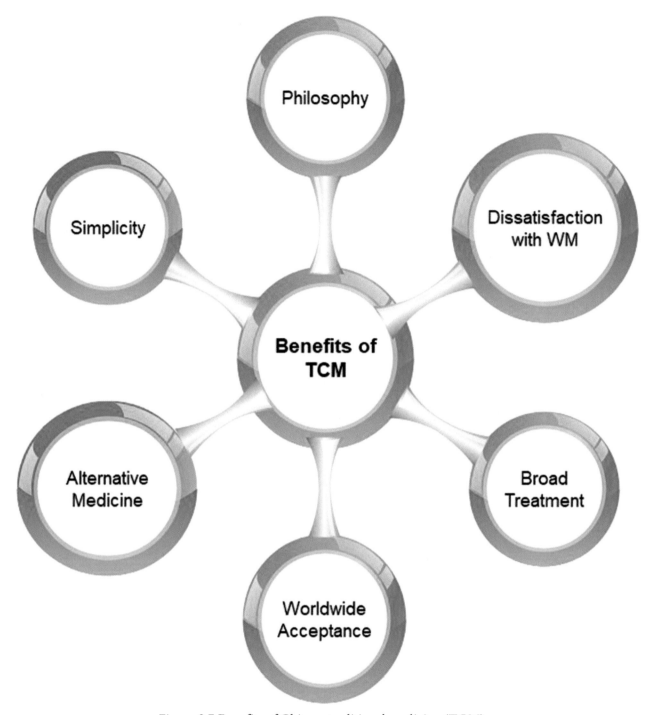

Figure 2.7 Benefits of Chinese traditional medicine (TCM).

2.9 CHALLENGES

Some of the herbs used in Chinese medicine can interact with drugs and have serious side effects. The pharmacology of TCM remains poorly understood. It is expedient for Chinese government and industry to increase the investments in developing TCM. Other challenges include the following [19-21]:

- *Skepticism:* In spite of the widespread use of TCM, there is skepticism about its true efficacy. A number of factors contribute to this skepticism. They can be potentially unsafe for people with some medical conditions. Critics argue that TCM was a pseudoscience that should be abolished in public healthcare.

- *Misapplication:* For most people, it is hard to recognize different Chinese herbs and how to use them. Lack of adequate knowledge of the Chinese herbs may cause misuse of the herbs. Some patients consume TCM products without consulting with their primary physician.

- *Toxicity:* Since TCM has become popular in the Western world, there are increasing concerns about the potential toxicity of many traditional Chinese medicine including plants, animal parts, and mineral. Traditional herbal medicines are sometimes contaminated with toxic heavy metals, which can inflict serious health risks to consumers.

- *Complexity:* Any disease will manifest itself differently in different patients. This is due to the complex interactions between a patient's environment and numerous physiological and pathological factors. Consequently, patient diagnosis and treatment in real-world settings are difficult, requiring precision medicine. It appears TCM follows complicated concepts and rules, making it very difficult to explain and prove in modern scientific means.

- *Scientific Evidence:* TCM needs rigorous, scientific evaluation to demonstrate its efficacy. In most cases, there is no rigorous scientific evidence to know whether TCM methods work as claimed. The herbs recommended by traditional Chinese practitioners in the US are not regulated or allowed to pass through rigorous scientific evidence of their effectiveness. The US Food and Drug Administration (FDA) will not allow medical practice without verifiable scientific evidence. The standards for evaluating Western medicine, which centers on "evidence-based medicine," are not suitable for testing TCM.

- *Quality:* The quality of the herbal product has become a critical issue for research and development. If the composition of the final herbal product is variable, then there is a strong possibility that the patient may be underdosed or overdosed.

- *TCM and Western Medicine:* The two medical practices have different viewpoints about etiology and pathology and thus different diagnostic methodologies. In Western medicine (WM), a disease is thought to develop as a result of one or more pathogenetic factors. In TCM, a disease is a common product of both pathogenetic factors and maladjustments in the body. The two systems of TCM and Western medicine need not clash. They are complimentary, taking advantage of the best features of each system and compensating for certain weaknesses in each.

- *Standardization:* The standards of evaluating Western medicine are not suitable for testing TCM.

These challenges are illustrated in Figure 2.8.

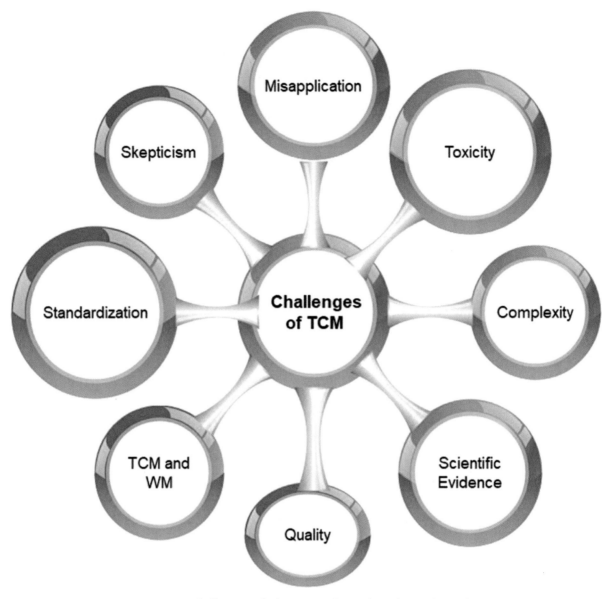

Figure 2.8 Challenges of Chinese traditional medicine (TCM).

2.10 CONCLUSION

The traditional Chinese medicine (TCM) thrives in the mainland China and is also widely used in Hong Kong, China, Taiwan, China, Japan, and South Korea. It is an integral part of Chinese culture and history. It has emerged as a means of maintaining good health and treating diseases in Chinese communities and has been adopted recently by other nations. It may be regarded as the crystallization of the ancient Chinese people's experience in their fight against diseases. There has been increased global interest in TCM. Increased side effects, lack of curative treatment for several chronic diseases, high cost of new drugs, and emerging diseases are some reasons for renewed public interest in traditional medicines [5]. With development of Chinese nation, TCM is also constantly improving.

Although rigorous scientific evidence of its effectiveness is limited, TCM has become more popular in the Western world. Governments and individuals are becoming more open to TCM practices and are considering them as an integrated part of health service delivery.

TCM is being taught in China and outside China at different levels. Students can learn how to practice traditional Chinese medicine. More information about TCM can be found in the books in [22 -47] and the following journals devoted to it:

- *The American Journal of Chinese Medicine*
- *Journal of Traditional Chinese Medicine*
- *Journal of Traditional Chinese Medical Sciences*
- *Chinese Journal of Integrative Medicine*
- *Chinese Medicine and Culture,*
- *Journal of Herbal Medicine*
- *Journal of Integrative Medicine*
- *Journal of Ethnopharmacology.*
- *Journal of Alternative and Complementary Medicine*
- *Advances in Traditional Medicine*
- *Traditional Medicine and Modern Medicine*

REFERENCES

[1] M. N. O. Sadiku, T. J. Ashaolu, and S. M. Musa, "Traditional Chinese medicine,: A primer" *International Journal of Science, Environment and Technology,* vol. 8, no. 1, 2019, pp. 20-25.

[2] H. Beinfield and E. Korngold, "Chinese traditional medicine: An introductory overview," *Alternative Therapies,* vol. 1, no. 1, March 1995, pp. 44-52.

[4] "Traditional Chinese medicine," *Wikipedia,* the free encyclopedia
https://en.wikipedia.org/wiki/Traditional_Chinese_medicine

[6] "Kampo, the elements of traditional Japanese medicine," June 2018,
https://elementaljapan.com/2018/06/25/kampo-the-elements-of-traditional-japanese-medicine/

[7] B. Patwardha et al., "Ayurveda and traditional Chinese medicine: A comparative overview," *Advance Access Publication,* vol. 2, no. 4, October 2005, pp. 465–473, 2005.

[8] "What is TCM?"
https://www.tcmworld.org/what-is-tcm/

[9] "Traditional Chinese medicine: In depth,"
https://nccih.nih.gov/health/whatiscam/chinesemed.htm

[10] X. Min et al., "A database on treating drug addiction with traditional Chinese medicine," *Addiction,* vol. 102, 2006, pp. 282–288.

[11] T. P. Fan et al. (eds.), "The art and science of traditional medicine Part 1: TCM Today – A case for integration," *Science,* vol. 346, 2014.

[12] L. Ives, "Can acupuncture help menopause symptoms?'
March 2019, https://www.bbc.com/news/health-47279032

[13] "6 Traditional Chinese medicine techniques,"
https://www.practicalpainmanagement.com/patient/treatments/alternative/6-traditional-chinese-medicine-techniques

[14] C. Ling, X. Yue, and C. Ling, "Three advantages of using traditional Chinese medicine to prevent and treat tumor," *Journal of Integrative Medicine,* vol. 12, no. 4, July 2014, pp. 331-335.

[15] X. Q. Hou et al., "Evidence from the randomized controlled trials of traditional Chinese medicine compound in treating Alzheimer's disease," *Proceedings of the IEEE/ACM International Conference on Advances in Social Networks Analysis and Mining*, 2014, pp. 752-757.

[16] T. Efferth et al., "From traditional Chinese medicine to rational cancer therapy," *TRENDS in Molecular Medicine,* vol.13, no..8, July 2007, pp. 353-361.

[17] W. Xu et al., "Prospects of a comprehensive evaluation system for traditional Chinese medicine services," *Journal of Integrative Medicine*, vol. 15, no. 6, November 2017, pp. 426-432.

[18] C. Ling, X. Yue1, and C. Ling, "Three advantages of using traditional Chinese medicine to prevent and treat tumor," *Journal of Integrative Medicine,* vol.12, no.4, July 2014, pp. 331-335.

[19] K. D. Moudgil and B. M. Berman, "Traditional Chinese medicine: Potential for clinical treatment of rheumatoid arthritis," *Expert Review of Clinical Immunology,* vol. 10, no. 7, 2014, pp. 819-822.

[20] W. Lv, J. H. Piao, and J. G. Jiang, "Typical toxic components in traditional Chinese medicine," *Expert Opinion on Drug Safety,* vol. 11, no. 6, 2012, pp. 985-1002.

[21] W. Y. Jiang, "Therapeutic wisdom in traditional Chinese medicine: A perspective from modern science," *TRENDS in Pharmacological Sciences,* vol. 26,no.11, November 2005, pp. 558-563.

[22] Z. Liu and L. Liu (eds.), *Essentials of Chinese Medicine.* Springer, volumes 1 and 2, 2009.

[23] H. Wang and B. Zhu (eds.), *Basic Theories of Traditional Chinese Medicine.* Singing Dragon, 2011.

[24] E. Hsu, *The Transmission of Chinese Medicine.* Cambridge University Press, 1999.

[25] Y. Xinrong et al. (eds.), *Encyclopedic Reference of Traditional Chinese Medicine.* Springer Science & Business Media, 2003.

[26] J. B. Li et al. *Traditional Chinese Medicine.* Beijing: People's Medical Publishing House, 2008.

[27] Z. Bing and W. Hongcai, *Diagnostics of Traditional Chinese Medicine.* Singing Dragon, 2010.

[28] G. Maciocia, *The Practice of Chinese Medicine.* New York: Churchill Livingstone, 1994.

[29] H. L. Wolfe, *The Successful Chinese Herbalist: How to Prescribe Correctly, Gain Patient Compliance, and Operate a Profitable Dispensary.* Boulder, CO: Blue Poppy Press, 2006.

[30] M. C. Kang, *Foundations of Traditional Chinese Medicine.* Create Space, 2010.

[31] T. A. Garran, *Western Herbs according to Traditional Chinese Medicine: A Practitioner's Guide.* Healing Arts Press, 2008.

[32] M. Wu, *Traditional Chinese Medicine: Herbal Formulas for Use in TCM with Differentiations of Symptoms.* Sun Garden Health Publisher, 2020.

[33] E.A. Poulin, *Traditional Chinese Medicine Curriculum Review: Pulling it all Together and Passing Exams.* CreateSpace Independent Publishing, 2016.

[34] L. Ursinus, *The Body Clock in Traditional Chinese Medicine: Understanding Our Energy Cycles for Health and Healing.* Earthdancer Books, 2020.

[35] Y. Ni, *Navigating the Channels of Traditional Chinese Medicine.* Complementary Medicine, 2004.

[36] V. Lo and M. Stanley-Baker (eds.), *Routledge Handbook of Chinese Medicine.* Routledge, 2022.

[37] A. Woods, *Chinese Herbal Medicine For Beginners: A Comprehensive Beginner's Guide of Natural Chinese Herbal Remedies for Faster Healing, Improved Wellness, and Boosting Energy.* Independently published, 2022.

[38] C. Chauhan, *Chinese Herbal Medicine for Beginners: Over 100 Remedies for Wellness and Balance.* Rockridge Press, 2020.

[39] G. Maciocia, *The Foundations of Chinese Medicine: A Comprehensive Text.* New York: Churchill Livingstone, 3rd edition, 2015.

[40] P. Chen and P. Xie. *History and Development of Traditional Chinese Medicine*. IOS Press, volume 1, 1999.

[41] M. Jiuzhang and G. Lei (eds.), *A General Introduction to Traditional Chinese Medicine*. Boca Raton, FL: CRC Press, 2009.

[42] B. Flaws and P. Sionneau, *The Treatment of Modern Western Medical Diseases with Chinese Medicine*. Boulder, CO: Blue Poppy Press, 2nd Edition, October 2005.

[43] Y. Xinrong (ed.), *Traditional Chinese Medicine: A Manual from A-Z*. Berlin: Springer-Verlag, 2003.

[44] S. Xutian (ed.), *Handbook of Traditional Chinese Medicine*. World Scientific, 3 volumes, 2014.

[45] Y. Zhang, Comprehensive Handbook of Traditional Chinese Medicine: Prevention & Natural Healing. Shanghai Press, 2020.

[46] Y. C. Lin and E. S. Z. Shen (eds.), *Acupuncture for Pain Management*. Springer, 2014.

[47] J. Aiyana, *Chinese Medicine & Healthy Weight Management*. Boulder, CO: Blue Poppy Press, 2007.

3

Traditional Indian Medicine

"Foolish the doctor who despises the knowledge acquired by the ancients."
-- Hippocrates

3.1 INTRODUCTION

Food is the main source of providing nutritional needs. The food security of any nation is directly related to the food and health security of its citizens. Health and illness have always been a primary concern of human beings. Every medical system aims to restore those who are ill to health. From ancient time, nature has bestowed incredible boons on mankind as it provides food, shelter, medicine, and animal resources to meet our needs. Folk or traditional medicine refers to diverse health practices, knowledge, and skills based on ancient indigenous experience that are used to maintain health as well as to cure, diagnose, or prevent illness. Traditional medicine is still playing a vital role, especially in rural areas, and will always play an imperative role in global healthcare system [1].

The population of India is roughly 1.38 billion, with more than 70% of of the population living in rural or remote areas. In India, two parallel medical systems (modern and traditional) exist side by side. Modern medicine is evidence-based, while traditional medicine has not gone through critical evaluation. India is blessed with an ancient heritage of traditional Indian medicine (TIM), which relies on lifelong medication on which patients can depend. TIM remains one of the most ancient yet living traditions. It has a rich history of its effectiveness. It consists of six traditional medicinal systems: Ayurveda, Siddha, and Unani, Yoga, Naturopathy, and Homoeopathy. Of these six, Ayurveda is the most famous. Efforts to regulate TIM are ongoing because of the increasing renewed global interest in complementary and alternative medicines [2].

This chapter provides an overview of Ayurveda, the traditional Indian medicine. It begins by providing a brief history. It consider the six India traditional medicinal systems and focusses on the most popular system, Ayurveda. It presents some herbs used in Ayurveda. It discusses some of applications of Ayurveda. It addresses the globalization of TIM. It highlights the benefits and challenges of TIM. The last section concludes with comments.

3.2 BRIEF HISTORY OF AYURVEDA

India has a long history of traditional medicine with Ayurveda being the most representative. Indian civilization is one of the oldest heritages of mankind. Indian traditional medicinal system or Ayurveda is a one of the oldest traditional medicinal systems in the world. The Ayurvedic concept originated and developed in India between 2500 and 500 BC. It flourished throughout the Indian Middle Ages. The Arabian scholars and physicians under the patronage of Islamic rulers of many Arabian nations have played a great role in the development of this system. The Arabs were instrumental in introducing Unani medicine in India around 1350 AD. Unani medicine has its origin in Greece. The Arabic works derived from the Ayurvedic texts eventually also reached Europe by the 12th century.

During the period of colonial British rule of India, the practice of Ayurveda was neglected by the British Indian Government, in favor of Western medicine. After gaining independence from Britain in 1947, the traditional systems of medicine was revived. The government of India initiated measures to improve Ayurveda as one of the major health care systems. The traditional medical systems got official recognition and became a part of the Indian national health care system, with state hospitals for Ayurveda established across the nation to provide healthcare to the country's citizens. Government of India initiated a series of measures to improve the status of Ayurveda. A national policy for the development of Indian System of Medicine (ISM) was developed and many research centers were established [3].

It was in 1970 that India changed its pre-independence policy and recognized Ayurveda and other medical systems to promote the development of national health. Since then, a large number of Ayurveda hospitals and clinics have been established throughout the country, most of which are funded and managed by the national and state governments.

Beginning in the 1960s, Ayurveda has been advertised as alternative medicine in the Western world. In 1970 India changed its pre-independence policy and recognized Ayurveda and other medical systems. Ayurveda now has its own department for management. At the moment, there are more than 200 colleges which offer several courses leading to bachelor degree in Ayurvedic medicine. In the United States, the practice of Ayurveda is not licensed or regulated by any state [4].

3.3 INDIAN TRADITIONAL MEDICINAL SYSTEMS

As shown in Figure 3.1, India is well known for its six traditional medicinal systems: Ayurveda, Siddha, and Unani, Yoga, Naturopathy, and Homoeopathy. Of these traditional systems, Ayurveda is the most popular. The Indian Systems of Medicine (ISM) are often termed 'AYUSH' – an acronym based on Ayurveda, Yoga, Unani, Siddha, and Homoeopathy, the five major indigenous medical systems in the country.

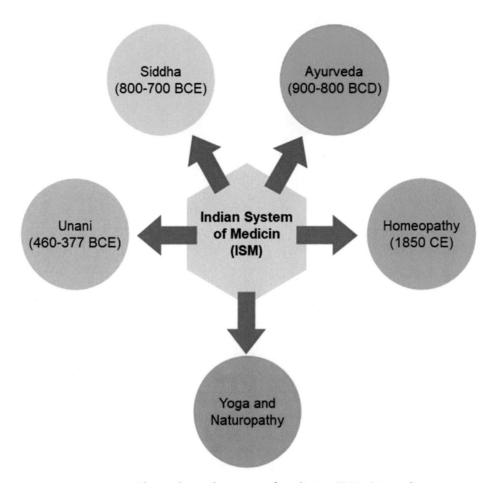

Figure 3.1 The traditional systems of medicine (TSMs) in India.

A separate ministry of Ayurveda, Yoga and Naturopathy, Unani, Siddha and Homeopathy (AYUSH) has been constituted under the government of India. These six traditional Indian medical systems are summarized as follows [5]:

- *Ayurveda:* For over 2000 years most of the Indian population have used Ayurveda as their major healthcare system. About 70 percent of rural population in India depends on the traditional Ayurvedic medicines. Ayurveda is not just a system of medicine, it is the science of life of the universe and is therefore universally applicable. It teaches us the science of life from a micro level to a macro level and helps us to maintain the equilibrium state of the body's elements. Ayurvedic medicines are not only used for primary healthcare in developing nations, they are also used in developed nations where conventional, modern medicines compete. The quality, safety, stability, and efficiency for Ayurveda products are now being investigated through research.

- *Siddha:* This is the oldest medical system in the world. Siddha system of medicine is settled since the ancient human civilization in India, around 10,000 BCE–4000 BCE. This practice of medicine is based on Saiva philosophy, one out of six branches of Hindu religion. The word "Siddha" indicates "holy harmony" or "attaining excellence" or "recognized fact" and the "Siddhars" were supernatural beings who obtain intellectual powers by constant practice of such type of medicine. The Siddha medicinal practice believes preserving the human well-being is crucial to succeeding the eternal bliss.

- *Unani:* The Unani system of medicine is a comprehensive medication. It originated in Greece, and later it was introduced in India by Arabs. It is based on the four conditions of living: as hot, sodden, frosty, and dry and four humors: namely, blood, yellow bile, dark bile, and mucus. Unani views the human body as made up of seven standards: Mizaj (temperaments), Anza (organs), Quo (resources), Arkan (components), Arawh (spirits), Aklath (humors), and Afal (capacities). Types of medications recommended in the Unani system of medicine are diet therapy, regimental treatment, and pharmaco-treatment. The Unani system extends great solutions for gastrointestinal, nervous disorders, and cardiovascular disease.

- *Homeopathy:* The term "homoeopathy" has been derived from Greek words. "Homois" which means similar and "pathos" which means suffering. Homeopathy is not an indigenous system; it came to India in the eighteenth century. It is a therapeutic technique that is based on two main principles: (1) "Like cures like;" a healthy individual would manifest the same symptom with the drug, that particular drug is the cure for the same illness; (2). "Infinite dilution;" therapeutic activity is enhanced by repeated dilution and succession. Homeopathy techniques essentially imply treating illnesses with cures. They have been polished since over 200 years in India and are now practiced throughout the world.

- *Yoga:* Yoga is a Sanskrit word. The word has changing interpretations yet is most usually comprehended. Yoga originated in India in ancient times. It is basically a physical, mental and spiritual practice, which deals with physical, mental, and spiritual condition of a person. Yoga explores preventive and curative aptitudes as a training exercise for people to improve mindfulness and calmness. As shown in Figure 3.2, yoga is about performing different poses for increasing your strength and flexibility [6]. Yoga centers are growing at a faster rate. Indian yoga has a huge following across India, China, and in the West. June 21 was declared as the International Day of Yoga by the United Nations General Assembly on December 11, 2014.

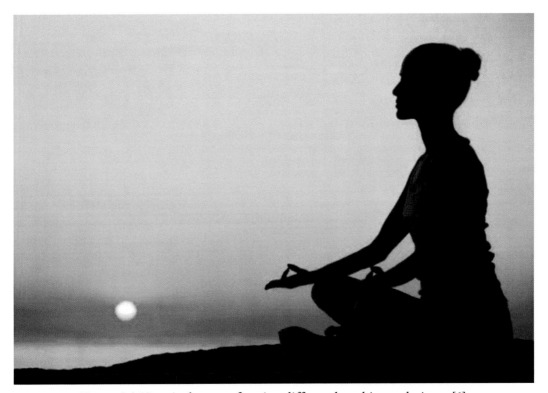

Figure 3.2 Yoga is about performing different breathing techniques [6].

3.4 AYURVEDIC SYSTEM

Ayurveda is a Sanskrit word that means "the wisdom of life" or "the knowledge of longevity." It is a compound of "ayus" meaning life or longevity and "veda" meaning deep knowledge or wisdom. Some also interpret Ayurveda to mean the science of life. It is the science of life of the universe. It takes into consideration physical, psychological, philosophical, ethical, and spiritual well being of people. Ayurveda is regarded not just as an ethnomedicine but it lays great importance on living in harmony with the nature. It lays great emphasis on the preservation of health. It emphasizes maintaining proper lifestyle in order to have positive health. American Indians regard traditional Indian medicine (TIM) as spirituality. Ayurveda is comparable to traditional Chinese medicine. Besides India, Ayurveda is also practiced in Sri Lanka.

Ayurvedic medicine is one of the world's oldest medical systems. It describes the beneficial, nonbeneficial, happy, and unhappy aspects of life. The practitioner of Ayurveda employs all five senses in diagnosis. He takes a careful note of the patient's internal physiological characteristics and mental disposition. He believes that everything is made of five cosmic elements: earth, fire, air, water, and ether, as illustrated in Figure 3.3 [7].

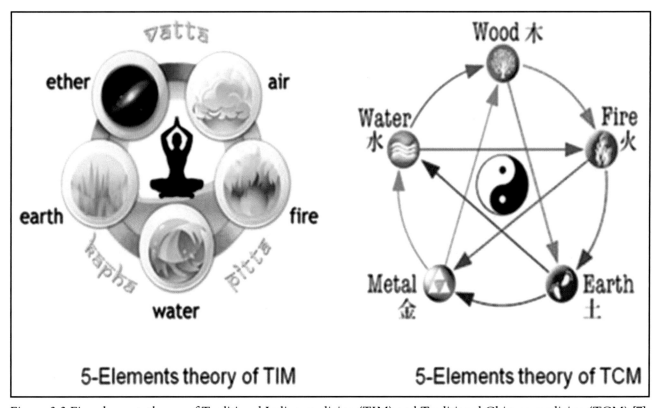

Figure 3.3 Five elements theory of Traditional Indian medicine (TIM) and Traditional Chinese medicine (TCM) [7].

Diagnosis and treatment tend to be human characteristics rather than the disease itself [3].

- *Ayurveda's Diagnosis:* Ayurveda divides diseases into two categories: those suitable for medical or surgical treatment, and those causing mental or physical pain. In traditional Indian society, diagnosis is often carried out by considering the patient as a whole object. The practitioner of Ayurveda considers details of personal, social, economic, and environmental situation of the patient. He asks detailed questions about the history of the illness and about such things as the patient's taste, smell, and dreams. The medicine man is a person of much power and he is regarded as healer, priest, advisor, and arbitrator. He works under the guidance of a guardian spirit and his pronouncements are backed by spiritual authority. A man selling traditional Indian medicine on a street in Mumbai, India is shown in Figure 3.4 [8]. It is usually presumed that the knowledge of Ayurveda is given by the gods of a different world. Ayurveda is based on folklore. Curing rituals are mostly private [9].

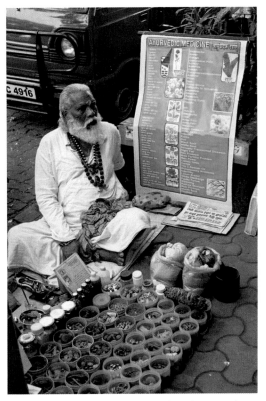

Figure 3.4 A man selling traditional Indian medicines [8].

Ayurveda has eight ways to diagnose illness [10]: Nadi (pulse), Mootra (urine), Mala (stool), Jihva (tongue), Shabda (speech), Sparsha (touch), Druk (vision), and Aakruti (appearance). The medicine can treat fever, cough, diarrhea, dropsy, seizures, diabetes, tumors, asthma, cancer, anemia, heart disease, leprosy, boils, skin disorders, ulcers, gout, diseases of the eye, headache, and wound. The treatment prescribed is designed to restore the balance of disturbed humors through regulating diet, correcting life-routine and behavior, and administration of drugs.

- *Ayurveda Treatment:* Ayurveda takes into consideration the actions of the drug in its entirety. The drugs used are mainly animals, minerals, and marine drugs. In clinical practice, the drugs used are single or compound. Indian herbal uses the oil extracted from herbs to remove toxins from the body and restore the body to a natural balance. Many factors must be considered when prescribing or taking Ayurvedic medicine. Ayurveda has timings for medication according to the patient's nature, disease, and the condition of disease and most medications are administered after food. Ayurvedic medicines exist in different formats such as liquids, powders, pastes, fermented products, tablets, and medicinal butters. The formats used depends on preparations' efficacy [11].

There are two divisions of Ayurveda: Swasthavritta and Athuravritta.. Within Ayurveda there are eight specialties [12]:

Kayachikitsa - internal medicine

Kaumarabhritya - paediatrics and gynaecology

Shalyatantra - surgery

Shalakyatantra - ophthalmology and otorihnolaryngyology

Grihachikitsa - psychiatry

Agatatantra - toxicology

Rasayanatantra - geriatrics / rejuvenation therapy

Vajeekaranatantra - sexology / virilification

3.5 HERBAL MEDICINE

Recently, the popularity of herbal medicine has increased worldwide for healthcare management. People from many developed and developing nations have been attracted toward traditional Indian herbal medicines. Traditional treatments include herbal medicines, dietary interventions, and massage. Ayurveda uses herbs, metals (e.g. gold, lead, mercury), organic matters, and minerals. India has a large diversity of plant species, which are the major source of drug in TIM. India is also the largest producer of medicinal herbs and is called as botanical garden of the world.

Plants are regarded as divine in origin and were worshipped as goddesses. The Indian subcontinent is a vast repository of medicinal plants that are used in traditional medical treatments. Plants are the primary ingredients of Ayurvedic drugs. These plant species are being explored with the modern scientific approaches for better leads in the healthcare. Herbal medicine includes herbs, herbal materials, and products. Medicinal plants are often used by traditional doctors to treat a variety of ailments and symptoms such as fever, cold, headache, ulcer, diabetes, and cancer. Figure 3.5 shows the percentage of plants used in different systems of medicines in India [7].

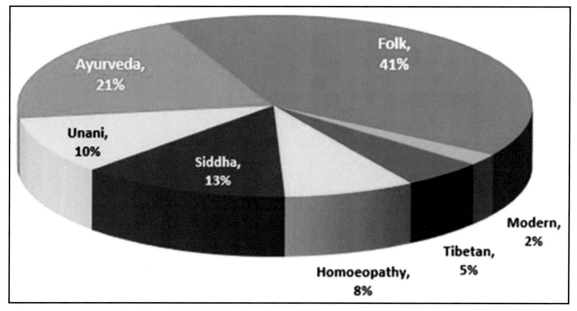

Figure 3.5 The percentage of plants used in different systems of medicines in India [5].

A lot of studies have been done on medicinal plants used in Indian traditional medicine. These include publications providing names of drugs used in particular type of disease conditions. Over 9,500 wild species used by tribal groups for meeting various needs have been recorded so far. Research effort in traditional medicine has focused mainly on medicinal plants. The World Health Organization (WHO) lists 21,000 plants used for medicinal purposes all over the world.

The following are some of the Indian medical plants [13,14]:

- *Holy basil:* This plant is native to the Indian subcontinent and has a place within the home of every Hindu. It is used for herbal tea.
- *Coriander:* This is grown for its leaves and used in cuisines throughout the world. It is most traditionally used in Indian cooking. It is shown in Figure 3.6 [13].

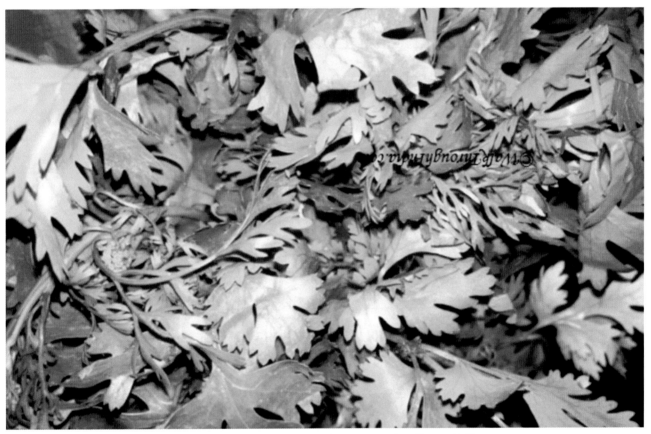

Figure 3.6 A typical India plant, coriander/dhania [13].

- *Spearmint:* This is the main ingredient of the summer drinks of India Its leaves are also used for spearmint tea.
- *Ajwain:* This originated in India and the leaves are used in traditional Ayurvedic medicine for stomach disorders.
- *Aloe Vera:* This has many medicinal uses, mostly found in beverages, cosmetics, and lotion.
- *Tinospora Cordifolia:* This is one of the most divine herb of India and a must use Indian medicine without causing any harmful effects.
- *Mustard:* This plant is from the foothills of the Himalaya in India and mustard seeds are used as a Indian spice.
- *Curry Tree:* This is native to India and curry leaves are used in most of the Indian dishes.

- *Indian Sorrel:* This leave is used in Ayurveda. The Indian herb is used in digestive disorders and diarrhea.
- *Boswellia:* This is also known as Indian frankincense. It is known for its easily recognizable spicy aroma. It may help prevent oral infections and fight gingivitis. It can accelerate menstrual flow and may induce miscarriage in pregnant women.
- *Triphala:* This is a popular remedy that may help reduce joint inflammation, improve digestion, and promote oral health. It contains powerful anti-inflammatory compounds that may help protect against certain cancers and other chronic diseases.
- Brahmi: This is a herb believed to lower inflammation, improve brain function, and reduce symptoms of attention deficit hyperactivity disorder (ADHD), such as inattention, impulsivity, poor self-control, and restlessness.
- *Cumin:* This is a spice commonly used to add flavor to meals. It is very dense in iron, providing almost 20% of your daily iron in one teaspoon. It may improve risk factors for type 2 diabetes and heart disease, and perhaps offer some protection against foodborne infection.
- *Turmeric:* This is the spice that gives curry its yellow color. Curcumin, its main compound, may help reduce inflammation and improve heart and brain health.
- *Licorice Root:* This is a spice that may help reduce inflammation and protect against various infections. It may also treat digestive problems and relieve skin irritations.
- *Gotu Kola:* This is a herb that may help boost memory and reduce stress, anxiety, and depression, as well as improve a variety of skin conditions.
- *Bitter Melon:* This is a spice that may help lower blood sugar levels and boost insulin secretion. It may also reduce bad cholesterol levels.
- *Cardamom*: This is a spice that may lower blood pressure, improve breathing, and potentially help stomach ulcers heal.
- *Bacopa monnieri:* This is a herbal remedy that grows in wet, tropical environments. It may help reduce stress and anxiety by elevating mood and reducing cortisol levels.

This list is not exhaustive but typical. Some of these herbs are available in many forms (tablets, powder, capsule, etc.) but most commonly taken in capsule form. Some can be purchased at health food stores and online.

3.6 APPLICATIONS

India has become the largest exporter of medicinal plants, plant drugs, and value-added products (e.g., essential oils, gum) in the world. Ayurvedic medications have been successfully used for the treatment of bronchial asthma, heart disease and hyperlipidaemia. Hindu surgeons operate on cataracts by couching, or displacing the lens to improve vision. The following are popular uses of TIM.

- *Drugs:* In India, about 70% of modern drugs are found in natural resources. At least 44% of India's plant resources can be developed into drugs.

Pharmaceutical companies have started to manufacture Ayurvedic and other forms of traditional medicines on a large scale. There are more than 8500 manufacturers of Ayurvedic drugs in the country. To aid marketing, India's traditional pharmaceutical manufacturers have always been in line with international thinking and have explored the international market. Ayurvedic drugs are marketed in various forms: classical forms (tablets, powder, decoction, medicated oil, medicated ghee, fermented products) and modern drug presentation forms like capsules, lotions, syrups, ointments, liniments, creams, granules etc. Ayurvedic drugs are marketed in various forms. They are available in both classical forms (tablets, powder, decoction, medicated oil, medicated ghee, fermented products) and modern drug presentation forms like capsules, lotions, syrups, ointments, liniments, creams, granules etc. [15]. Ayurveda medicine can protect and promote health by promoting longevity and preventing or delaying the aging process. It can also be effective in the treatment of some chronic diseases, such as cardiovascular diseases, cancer, fever, and inflammatory diseases, and kidney diseases.

- *Diabetes:* This is a chronic disorder of carbohydrate, fat, and protein metabolism. It is a major crippling disease in the world leading to huge economic losses. More than 300 million people of the world are suffering from this chronic disease. Diabetes is often characterized by post prandial blood sugar levels. Studies conducted in India in the last decade have highlighted that not only is the prevalence of diabetes high but also that it is increasing rapidly in the urban population. Patients of diabetes either do not make enough insulin or their cells do not respond to insulin. Diabetes is categorized into two types. Type I diabetes (insulin dependent) is caused due to insulin insufficiency because of lack of functional beta cells. Type II diabetes (insulin independent) are unable to respond to insulin and can be treated with dietary changes, exercise, and medication. As a multifactorial disease, diabetes demands a multiple therapeutic approach. There are many herbal drug remedies and plants that can used in the treatment of diabetes. For example, diabeta, a formulation of Ayurvedic Cure, is safe and effective in managing diabetes as a single agent supplement to synthetic anti-diabetic drugs [16].
- *Cancer:* Cancer cells possess the ability to escape apoptosis by various ways. The aim of anticancer agents is to trigger the apoptosis signaling system in these cancer cells while disturbing their proliferation. A large number of medicinal plants and their purified constituents have shown beneficial therapeutic potentials. The anticancer property of medicinal plants is used in the traditional Indian medicine system for effective anticancer drug with minimal side effects [17].

Other diseases that TIM can care include fever, cough, diarrhea, dropsy, seizures, diabetes, tumors, asthma, cancer, anemia, heart disease, leprosy, boils, skin disorders, ulcers, gout, diseases of the eye, headache, wound, bronchial asthma, rheumatoid arthritis, ischemic heart disease, and COVID-19, among other illnesses.

3.7 GLOBALIZATION OF AYURVEDA

Ayurvedic medicine has enriched almost all medical systems in the world. Global acceptance of Ayurveda is increasing and demand for medicinal plants from India is in upsurge. TIM has gained steady international demand over the years. Ayurveda has spread around the world. Today, Ayurvedic drugs are used as food supplements in many places like US, Europe, India, and Japan. In many parts of the world, several physicians practice Ayurveda [15]. Several modern medical practitioners are increasingly recommending alternative remedies to patients when modern medicines fail to work or when it has more side effects.

Drug combination treatment is increasingly applied in many areas in medicine. The World Health Organization (WHO) has also recognized the importance of traditional medicine in developing countries.

The Indian traditional techniques of cure like Yoga, massages, and herbal therapy are gaining popularity in wellness industry. Ayurvedic treatments are usually undergone alongside and/or after conventional medical approaches. India has consistently promoted the integration of Indian Systems of Medicine (ISM) into the country's official health system, health policies, and programs. The integration of ISM with allopathic medicine is illustrated in Figure 3.7 [18].

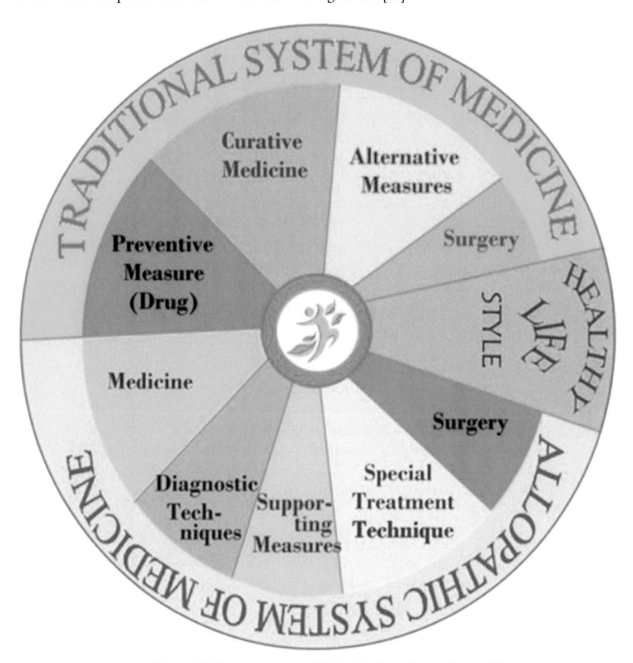

Figure 3.7 The integration of ISM with allopathic medicine [18].

3.8 BENEFITS

Nutrition is a basic human need. Dietary supplements and herbal remedies are popular complementary products people take. Herbal products are popularly known for their nutritional supplements. Traditional Indian Medicine (or Ayurveda) is among the well known global traditional systems of medicine and it is becoming increasingly popular. It is useful not only for the practitioners but also for housewives. It emphasizes diet, exercise, yoga, and meditation. Coupled with Indian medicine's thousands of years of clinical experience in using herbal medicine, this gives the country the opportunity to become the world's largest herbal manufacturer. TIM is gaining a multidimensional view into healthcare and health delivery among diverse groups including marginalized and indigenous populations. The traditional healing practices are respected by IHS employees in all our services and programs.

Other benefits include the following [19,20]:

- *Low Cost:* Inequities in the accessibility, availability, and affordability of modern healthcare make herbal drugs more popular in rural and remote areas. Plant-based medicines are well acknowledged for their economic importance.
- *Trust:* High cost for medical treatments, unsatisfactory treatment, and mistrust of people in current healthcare system signify the imperfection of modern medicinal system. These factors are the major reasons people have trust in the traditional medicine. The Indian traditional medicinal system provides strong evidence for their effectiveness and the rationale for why people continue to trust traditional knowledge.
- *Personalized Medicine:* Delivery of medicines is done in a personalized manner. The traditional healer performs a thorough examination of diseased individual and selects appropriate medicine in appropriate dosage for the patient.
- *Spiritual Healing:* Traditional Indian medicine (TIM) is regarded as spirituality. TIM holds that the practice is intended to restore balance and instill better health through consciousness and the connection between body, mind, and spirit. The aim is to achieve a better quality of life and health in all areas of life and prevent disease rather than treating it. It employs a holistic approach that combines diet, exercise, and lifestyle changes
- *Alternative to Western Medicine (WM):* Traditional medical practices are adjuncts or alternatives to Western medical approaches. The majority of Indians use Ayurvedic medicine exclusively or combined with conventional Western medicine. It is a well-known fact that traditional medicines supplement modern medicine in meeting the global healthcare needs in India, Southeast Asia, and the rest of the world.
- *Global Acceptance:* In nations beyond India, Ayurveda practices have been integrated in general wellness applications. The concepts of proper lifestyles and dietary habits followed in Ayurveda can be adopted to different nations. Indian traditional medicine has always played important role in meeting the global healthcare needs. It will play major role in future. For example, Ayurvedic drugs are used as food supplements in US, Europe, and Japan.

These benefits are displayed in Figure 3.8.

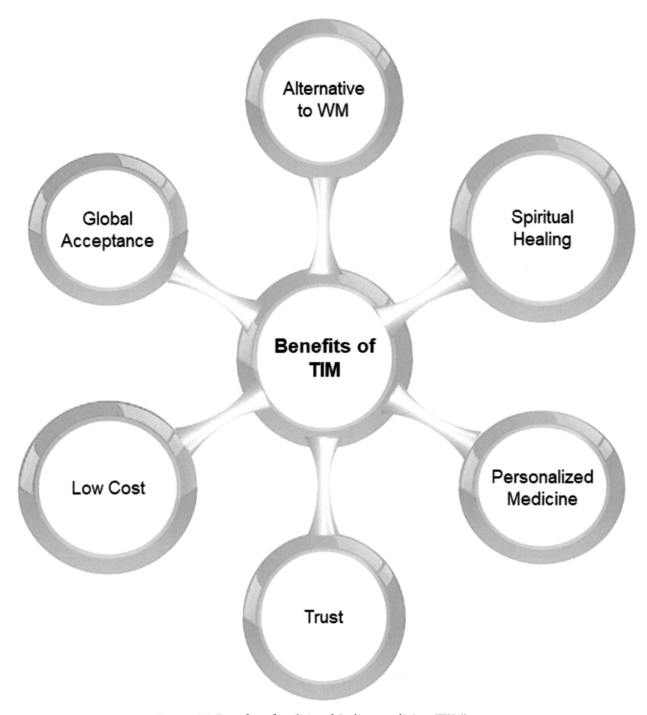

Figure 3.8 Benefits of traditional Indian medicine (TIM).

3.9 CHALLENGES

Evidence-based or scientific studies on the efficacy and safety of traditional Indian medicines are limited. The ancient wisdom in Indian traditional medical practices (Ayurveda, Siddha, Unani, and homeopathy) are still not fully explored. The major ingredients in most medical products are not clearly stated. TIM has taken only limited steps to scientifically validate the efficacy of its drugs. Today, Ayurveda is considered pseudoscientific. The practice of Ayurveda is not licensed by any state in the US and most Ayurvedic products are marketed without having been approved by the FDA. Other challenges of Ayurveda include the following [21,22]:

- *Scientific Evidence:* No significant scientific evidence has shown effectiveness of Ayurvedic medicine for the treatment of any disease. There are not enough well-controlled clinical trials and systematic research reviews to prove that the approaches are beneficial. Evidence-based studies on the efficacy and safety of Ayurveda are limited.
- *Promotion:* The promotion of traditional herbal medicine still faces many challenges, especially in developed nations. For successful promotion of TIM, these problems must be addressed [18]: (1) Quality issues, (2) quality control issues, (3) lack of regulation, (4) need for clinical trial, (5) research and development, (6) unethical practice, (7) protecting the medicinal plants.
- *Toxicity:* Ayurvedic products can be toxic. The products have been found to contain levels of lead, mercury, and/or arsenic that exceeded the standards for acceptable daily intake. In the US, Ayurvedic products are regulated as dietary supplements and are not expected to meet the same safety and effectiveness standards as conventional medicines.
- *Side Effects:* Approaches used in Ayurvedic medicine, such as massage, special diets, and cleansing techniques may have side effects as well. Several patients who use traditional medicines for a long time develop serious adverse effects on liver and kidney. Therefore, each person should be educated about the associated side effects of medicines. It is also necessary to check with your doctor before adding any Ayurvedic supplements to your healthcare regiment.
- *Safety:* Safety of some herbal products has been questioned. Traditional medicines may contain some ingredients that are no longer useful and can lead to side-effects. Therefore, safety is a major concern for TIM. Right quality of ingredients and no adulteration are two aspects of safety evaluation. Major obstacle in integrating herbal medicine and modern medical practices is lack of scientific and clinical data proving their efficacy and safety. The US FDA warns that some Ayurvedic products are potentially harmful because they contain some metals.
- *Plagiarism:* Intellectual property protection is a major challenge in India. Due to a lack of attention and awareness of safeguarding intellectual rights, many traditional drug patents have been plagiarized. Unavailability of a reference in modern language contributes to this problem.
- *Regulation:* The content and quality of traditional products are not regulated. In the US, regulations do not yet require that dietary supplement manufacturers adhere to standard manufacturing practices. So the quality of traditional products is not guaranteed,
- *Drug Standardization*: A major challenge with Ayurvedic medicines is the lack of drug standardization, information, quality control, and close monitoring. It is important to know the active component which will help to analyze therapeutic efficacy of the product and to standardize it.
- *Extinction of Plants:* The threat of extinction of certain species of plants and herbs is envisaged due the destruction of jungles, the greater demand for raw materials for increased manufacture of traditional medicinal preparations, and the lack of organized cultivation of medicinal plants.

These challenges are illustrated in Figure 3.9. The promotion and globalization of Indian traditional medicine will entail a more realistic and strong approach to overcome the difficulties.

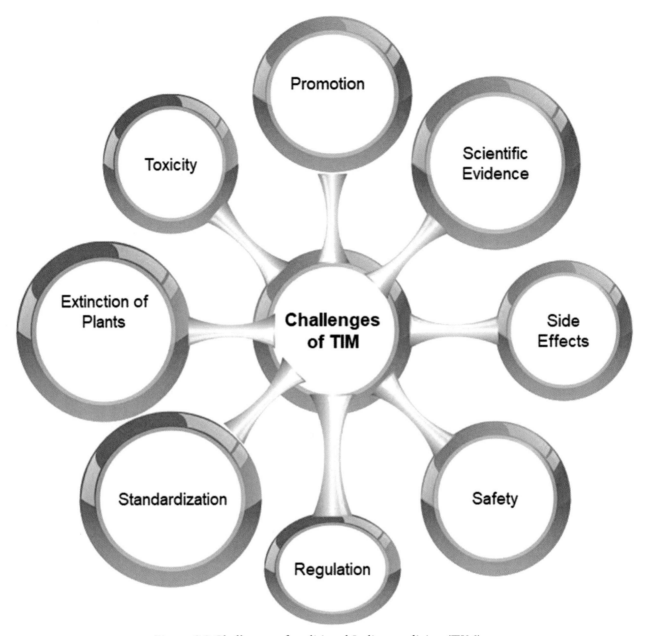

Figure 3.9 Challenges of traditional Indian medicine (TIM).

3.10 CONCLUSION

In India, two parallel systems of medicine (modern and traditional) operate side by side.

Traditional Indian medicine (TIM) refers the diverse health practices and approaches which are related to the beliefs and spiritual remedies. Although India has a number of traditional systems of medicine, Ayurveda is the most popular. Ayurveda is an Indian system of life sciences, documented and practiced since 1500 BCE. At the moment, Ayurveda is practiced across India and beyond, especially by those in rural or remote areas.

Ayurveda is one of the few medical systems developed in ancient times that is still widely practiced in modern times. It focuses on the management, education, regulation, development, and growth of Indian medicine in India and abroad. It basically includes perspectives of ceremonies, religion, practices, and medicine. It is a vast area of study that has been investigated in many ways. There is a trend towards increased usage of medicines used in traditional Indian systems especially those which are based on herbal products.

The California College of Ayurveda (CCA) provides the most comprehensive curriculum on Ayurveda in the United States. This state-approved program is designed for developing students for a career in restoring the natural balance of body, mind, and spirit with the wisdom of Ayurveda [23]. More information about Indian traditional medicine can be obtained from the books [24–40] and the following related journals:

- *Journal of Herbal Medicine*
- *Journal of Integrative Medicine*
- *Journal of Alternative and Complementary Medicine*
- *Journal of Traditional and Complementary Medicine*
- *Advances in Traditional Medicine*
- *Traditional Medicine and Modern Medicine*
- *Alternative and Complementary Therapies*
- *Journal of Evidence-Based Complementary & Alternative Medicine*

REFERENCES

[1]   S. Sen et al., "Indian traditional medicinal systems, herbal medicine, and diabetes," in S. Sen, R. Chakraborty, and B. De, *Diabetes Mellitus in 21*[st] *Century.* Singapore: Springer, 2016, pp. 125-151.

[2]   M. N. O. Sadiku, T. J. Ashaolu, and S. M. Musa, "Traditional Indian medicine," *International Journal of Trend in Scientific Research and Development*, vol. 3, no. 2, Jan.-Feb. 2019, pp. 321-322.

[3]   Y. Shi, C. Zhang, and X. Li, "Traditional medicine in India," *Journal of Traditional Chinese Medical Sciences,* vol. 8, supplement 1, November 2021, pp. S51-S55.

[4]   Y. S. Jaiswal and L. L. Williams, "A glimpse of Ayurveda – The forgotten history and principles of Indian traditional medicine," *Journal of Traditional and Complementary Medicine*, vol. 7, no. 1, January 2017,pp. 50-53.

[5]   P. P. Adhikari and S. H. Paul, "History of Indian traditional medicine: A medical inheritance," *Asian Journal of Pharmaceutical and Clinical Research,* vol. 11, no. 1, 2018, pp. 421-426.

[6]   "How to perform: 3 most common yoga breathing exercises," August 2021,
        https://timesofindia.indiatimes.com/life-style/health-fitness/fitness/how-to-perform-3-most-common-yoga-breathing-exercises/photostory/72400480.cms

[7]   S. F. Elahee, H. Mao, and X. Shen, "Traditional Indian medicine and traditional Chinese medicine: A comparative overview," *Chinese Medicine and Culture*, vol. 2, no. 3, 2019, pp. 105-113.

[8]   M. Williamson, "Traditional Indian medicine seller,"
        https://fineartamerica.com/featured/traditional-indian-medicine-seller-mark-williamson.html

[9]   M. E. Joy, "Traditional medicine at an Indian reserve," *Masters Thesis,* Michigan State University, 1989.

[10]   "Ayurveda," *Wikipedia*, the free encyclopedia
        https://en.wikipedia.org/wiki/Ayurveda

[11]   S. Kumar, G. J. Dobos, and T. Rampp, "The significance of Ayurvedic medicinal plants," *Journal of Evidence-Based Complementary & Alternative Medicine,* vol. 22, no. 3, 2017, pp. 494-501.

[12] Botanic Gardens Conservation International, "The teaching of Indian traditional medicine," https://www.bgci.org/education/1686

[13] "10 Indian medicinal plants to grow at your house," http://www.walkthroughindia.com/nursery/10-indian-medicinal-plants-to-grow-at-your-house/

[14] "12 Powerful Ayurvedic herbs and spices with health benefits," https://www.healthline.com/nutrition/ayurvedic-herbs

[15] B. Ravishankar and V. J. Shukla, "Indian systems of medicine: A brief profile," *African Journal of Traditional, Complementary and Alternative Medicines,* vol. 4, no. 3, 2007, pp. 319 – 337.

[16] M. Modak et al., "Indian herbs and herbal drugs used for the treatment of diabetes," *Journal of Clinical Biochemistry and Nutrition,* vol. 40, no. 3, May 2007, pp. 163–173.

[17] A. Baskar et al., "In vitro antioxidant and antiproliferative potential of medicinal plants used in traditional Indian medicine to treat cancer," *Redox Report,* vol. 17, no. 4, 2012, pp. 145-156.

[18] S. Sen and R. Chakraborty, "Revival, modernization and integration of Indian traditional herbal medicine in clinical practice: Importance, challenges and future," *Journal of Traditional and Complementary Medicine,* vol. 7, 2017, pp. 234-244.

[19] "Toward the integration and advancement of herbal medicine: A focus on traditional Indian medicine," https://www.dovepress.com/toward-the-integration-and-advancement-of-herbal-medicine-a-focus-on-t-peer-reviewed-fulltext-article-BTAT

[20] V. P. Gaonkar and K. Hullatti, "Indian traditional medicinal plants as a source of potent Anti-diabetic agents: A review," *Journal of Diabetes and Metabolic Disorders,* vol. 19, no. 2, September 2020, pp.1895-1908.

[21] R. Lodha and A. Bagga, "Traditional Indian systems of medicine," *Annals of the Academy of Medicine, Singapore,* vol. 29, no. 1, January 2000, pp. 37-41.

[22] P. B. Weragoda, "The traditional system of medicine in Sri Lanka," *Journal of Ethnopharmacology,* vol. 2, no. 1, March 1980, pp. 71-73.

[23] "Internationally recognized ayurvedic education," https://www.ayurvedacollege.com/california/

[24] D. Martin, *Ayurvedic Herbal Medicine for Beginners: More Than 100 Remedies for Wellness and Balance.* Rockridge Press, 2022.

[25] F. J. Ninivaggi, *Ayurveda: A Comprehensive Guide to Traditional Indian Medicine for The West.* Rowman & Littlefield Publishers, 2010.

[26] L. Verotta, M. P. Macchi, and P. Venkatasubramanian (eds.), *Connecting Indian Wisdom and Western Science: Plant Usage for Nutrition and Health (Traditional Herbal Medicines for Modern Times).* Boca Raton, FL: CRC Press, 2015.

[27] M. S. Premila, *Ayurvedic Herbs: A Clinical Guide to the Healing Plants of Traditional Indian Medicine.* Psychology Press, 2006.

[28] C. P. Khare, *Indian Herbal Remedies: Rational Western Therapy, Ayurvedic, and Other Traditional Usage, Botany.* Springer Science & Business Media, 2004.

[29] J. S. Alter (ed.), *Asian Medicine and Globalization.* Philadelphia: University of Pennsylvania Press, 2005.

[30] L. A. Alvord, and E. C. V. Pelt, *The Scalpel and the Silver Bear. The First Navajo Woman Surgeon Combines Western Medicine and Traditional Healing.* Des Plaines, IL: Bantam Books, 1999.

[31] M .S. Premila, *Ayurvedic Herbs: A Clinical Guide to the Healing Plants of Traditional Indian Medicine.* Routledge, 2006.

[32] H. H. Rhyne, *Llewellyn's Complete Book of Ayurveda: A Comprehensive Resource for the Understanding & Practice of Traditional Indian Medicine.* Llewellyn Publications, 2017.

[33] P. Gonzales, *Traditional Indian Medicine: American Indian Wellness.* Kendall Hunt Publishing Company, 2017.

[34] R. K. Bhutiya, *Ayurvedic Medicinal Plants of India.* India, Scientific Publishers, volume 1,2011.

[35] E. J. Waring and M. Sheriff, *A Catalogue of Synonymes of the Indian Medicinal Plants, Products, and Organic Substances: Included in that Work, With Explanatory and Descriptive Remarks.* Asiatic Publishing House, 2 volumes, 2008.

[36] A. Chatterjee and S. C. Pakrashi, *Treatise on Indian Medicinal Plants.* Vedic Book, 6 volumes, 1997.

[37] N. Tandon and P. Sharma, *Quality Standards of Indian Medicinal Plants.* Indian Council of Medical Research, volume 13, 2015.

[38] N. Tandon, *Reviews on Indian Medicinal Plants.* Indian Council of Medical Research, volume 17, 2017.

[39] V. K. Gupta, *Traditional and Folk Herbal Medicine: Recent Researches.* Daya Publishing House, volume 2, 2014.

[40] S. Sen and R. Chakraborty, *Herbal Medicine in India : Indigenous Knowledge, Practice, Innovation and Its Value.* Singapore: Springer Verlag, 2019.

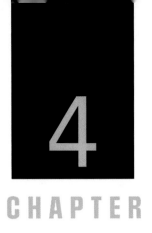

Japanese Traditional Medicine

"The practice of medicine is an art, based on science." – William Osler

4.1 INTRODUCTION

True medicine should target the overall health of every human being not only as a science but also as an art. Our health is our most important asset. In ancient times disease was regarded as sent by the gods or caused by evil spirits. Prevention, diagnosis, and treatment were based largely on religious practices, such as prayers, fasting, incantations, divination, and exorcism. Humans have used natural products, such as plants, animals, and microorganisms to prevent illnesses and treat diseases.

The Japanese have developed their own special medicine for treatment. Cultural contact between China and Japan has occurred since ancient times. Some Chinese medical works were introduced to Japan as early as the 4th or 5th Century A.D., coming first by way of Korea, introduced the concept of social medicine to Japan. Japanese colonialists propagandized the "benefits of modern civilization such as western medicine" and rejected the advantages of traditional medicine [1].

Kampo medicines have been used in Japan since the early Edo period (17th century). The medical practice is designed to heal the physical bodies of humans and animals with the aim of eradicating all ills in the world. Traditional Japanese medicine or Kampo is a diverse and dynamic form of medicine. Kampo practitioners often reflect on principles, treating patients of all ages and conditions. From maintaining wellbeing to the treatment of stubborn and chronic issues, they approach the health of patients with care and diligence. Japanese traditional medicines (JTM) have been mainly used to treat chronic diseases. The effectiveness of Kampo medicine in treating various diseases is attracting more and more attention in the Japanese medical system. They are increasingly recognized to have useful clinical applications in Japan and beyond. The World Health Organization (WHO) encourages the integration of traditional medicine into Western medicine. The two systems of medicine can be complementary, each strengthening the inadequacies of the other.

This chapter provides an introduction in Japanese traditional medicine, Kampo. It begins by briefly covering the history of Kampo. It discusses the concept of Kampo, its diagnosis, and treatment. It provides information on Japanese herbs. It presents some applications of Kampo. It highlights the benefits and challenges of Kampo. It covers global adoption of Kampo. The last section concludes with comments.

4.2 BRIEF HISTORY OF KAMPO

Kampo medicine has a history of nearly 1500 years in Japan. It is derived from traditional Chinese medicine (TCM) and consists of various herbal products. It evolved throughout history into a uniquely distinct form. The very beginning of Kampo was when Chinese medicine was brought into Japan bypassing the Korean peninsula in the 5th Century. As the Edo era began, Japan took a national isolation policy which blocked all contacts with nations that include China. During this period, Japan traditional medicine developed by integrating Japanese culture with the traditional Chinese medical practices. This was when the traditional Japanese medical practices started being called "kampo" to distinguish one from the other medical systems. Japan only grows 12% of Kampo herbs that the nation consumes, and the rest 80% of herbs are imported from China [2].

Western medicine was introduced to Japan by the Portuguese around 1590. The biggest boost to Western medicine in Japan came with the introduction of smallpox vaccination in 1849, when Kampo had no comparable disease prevention techniques. Kampo then went into a period of severe decline from 1868 to 1902 as the result of efforts by the Meiji government which only recognized the German or Western medical system. The Meiji government was not successful in eliminating Kampo because several Kampo physicians continued to promote the tradition. After 1902, Kampo experienced a gradual revival as it was no longer regarded as a potential threat to modernization.

When Japan was defeated in 1945, it took several years for the country and its industrial and social activities to recover. The medical doctors (including Kampo physicians) who had taken up the practice of Kampo formed the Japan Society for Oriental Medicine in 1950 with 98 members. With only slight modifications, it has been adopted also in Taiwan and exported from Taiwan to the West. Kampo was brought to Taiwan by Dr. Hong-yen Hsu, who later immigrated to the United States in the mid-seventies and introduced Kampo to America. Sun Ten established a factory to manufacture Kampo medicines in the US. Kampo in the West is becoming integrated into a broader system with the intention of combining effectively with modern (Western) medicine [3].

Today, Kampo is a distinctive, holistic practice that is Kampo widely practiced in Japan and is fully integrated into the Japanese modern national healthcare system. Although Kampo is based on traditional Chinese medicine, it is adapted to Japanese culture. What strongly influenced the practice of Kampo during the past 25 years was the formal recognition, by the Japanese Ministry of Health, of certain traditional Chinese herb formulas. Kampo is widely practiced today and is covered by national medical insurance.

4.3 CONCEPT OF JAPANESE TRADITIONAL MEDICINE

Traditional medicines use natural products and are of great importance. The word "traditional" implies the use of herbal medicines with substantial historical and indigenous use. Traditional medicine is also known as complementary and alternative, ethnic medicine, or folk medicine.

Traditional Japanese medicine can be classified into two groups: Japanese indigenous traditional medicine and Kampo. Kampo is the more popular. Kampo (also known as Chinese herbs or Sino-Japanese traditional medicine) is a traditional medical practice that originated from China and developed into its present form in Japan. It literally means the Han Method, referring to the herbal system of China that developed during the Han Dynasty. It came to Japan during the 7th through 9th centuries. The original medicine practice had also travelled into Korea and evolved into traditional Korean medicine. The underlying notion of Kampo is that the human body and mind are inseparable and a balance of physical and mental is essential for human health.

Kampo consists of three pillars: herbal medicine, acupuncture treatment, and physical care/curing. The physical care is the most important and demands that we eat, exercise, and sleep well. Kampo medicine is made of various natural resources such as plants, minerals, and animal parts. The combination of the ingredients produces different types of effects. It does not use endangered plants or animal products. Kampo is largely dependent on imported goods.

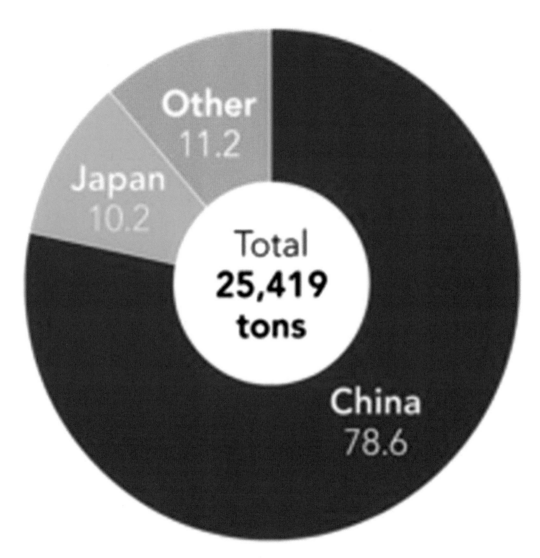

Figure 4.1 Origins of herbal medicine ingredients used in Japan (in percent) [4].

As shown in Figure 4.1, Japan only grows 10% of Kampo herbs consumed, while 78% of herbs are imported from China [4]. The current state of Kampo prescription is depicted in Figure 4.2 [2].

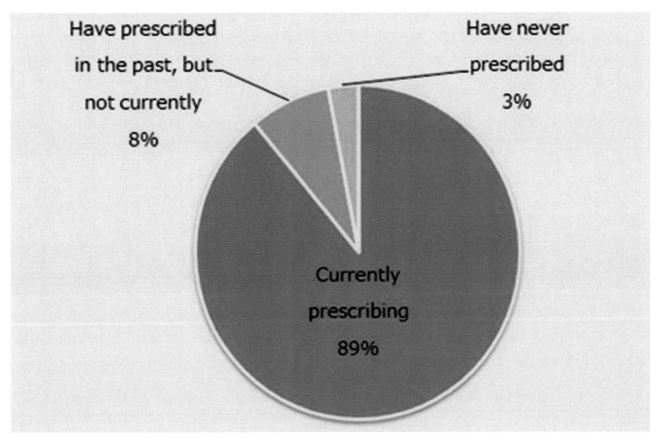

Figure 4.2 Current state of Kampo prescription [2].

The fundamental characteristics of Kampo include the following [5]:

- Kampo is a standardized multi-herb therapeutic tradition uniquely developed in Japan from ancient Chinese origins.
- Kampo therapies are personalized for the individual. Different formulas have been prescribed for patients with the same disease and diagnosis.
- Kampo therapies restore balance to the whole organism. Kampo understands the patients from a holistic perspective that emphasizes the importance of balancing and harmonizing the entire patient.
- Kampo practitioners do not share the Western concept of a mind–body split. Mind and body spirit are inseparable and interrelated in Kampo.
- Kampo practioners prioritize the subjective, qualitative, and intuitive aspects of medicine.

Traditional East Asian Medicine (TEAM) is a term that covers traditional medical systems from East Asia derived from early Chinese medical discourse. Traditional East Asian Medical (TEAM) practice systems exhibit much variation. Traditional East Asian Medicine (TEAM) uses a wide range of gentle and non-invasive treatment strategies to bring patients back to a state of health, vitality and wellness.

Yokukansan (YKS) is a traditional Japanese medicine collectively referred to as kampo in Japan. It is a herbal medicine that has recently been used to treat the behavioral and psychological symptoms of dementia, including aggressiveness, excitability, and hallucination. It has been approved in Japan as a remedy for neurosis, insomnia, and irritability in children. It has also been reported to improve behavioral and psychological symptoms in patients with various forms of dementia.

Maoto, a traditional Japanese medicine (Kampo), is widely used to treat upper respiratory tract infections, including influenza virus infection. The traditional Japanese herbal medicine Maoto is widely prescribed to treat symptoms of upper respiratory infections including influenza. Influenza, the disease targeted by Maoto, is a health issue of concern because it causes high morbidity and a high number of deaths. Maoto is an extract of four medicinal herbs [6].

4.4 KAMPO DIAGNOSIS AND TREATMENT

Among the Japanese practitioners with national licenses, only physicians are allowed to diagnose and treat patients according to various types of traditional medicine in addition to Western medical treatment [7].

- *Kampo Diagnosis*: This is made by listening to a patient's complaints and by performing a set of traditional examinations focusing on pulse, abdominal signs, and the appearance of the tongue. Japanese Kampo favors diagnostic methods that directly relate the symptoms to the therapy. Japanese physicians with limited education in Kampo diagnostics tend to apply the formulations according to conventional Western diagnoses. They arrive at diagnoses via four basic approaches [8]:

  1. Visual examination: Observation of the status of the face, tongue, skin, and behavior of the patient.
  2. Auditory examination: Auscultation of the patient speaking, sighing and wheezing, and examination of the patient's olfaction.
  3. Interview: Questions posed to the patient about the history of the illness.
  4. Tactile examination: Evaluation of the pulse and determination of abdominal status.

Diagnosis in the Kampo treatment involves the following steps [8]:

  1. Gathering data about symptoms to determine a diagnosis.
  2. Identifying the cause of the illness based on the theory underpinning traditional Chinese medicine (TCM), including the five-element theory described later.
  3. Determining the appropriate prescription based on the theory underpinning TCM. According to TCM, herbal prescriptions are based on imbalances in the viscera and bowels.

  - *Kamp Treatment:* Kampo incorporates Japanese herbal medicine as well as elements of acupuncture and moxibustion. It has been used extensively in both China and Japan for treatment of chronic liver diseases and other inflammatory conditions. Kampo has been used to alleviate the various symptoms of female menopause, improve memory impairment. It is commonly prescribed by Japanese traditional doctors or Kampo practitioners. Most of those doctors were gynecologists, urologists, and cardiologists.

Kampo medicine has been applied for disease prevention and maintenance of quality of life. It is administered using the Kampo theory, which involves analyzing three main indicators: Qi (well-being, energy, illness, vigor), blood, and water levels in the body. Abnormalities in these indicators would often lead to diseases. Symptoms of illnesses are often attributed to the product of disrupted, blocked or unbalanced Qi movement. For example, unbalanced Qi levels result in hair loss, osteoporosis, incontinence, cold legs, itching, and difficulty in hearing. The therapeutic objective of Kampo is to relieve symptoms and to restore harmony in bodily functions.

4.5 JAPANESE HERBS

Japanese herbal medicine deals primarily with the diagnosis and treatment of illness using herbs. Japanese doctors treat their patients using herbal medicine as well as the most advanced western medicine. Japanese herbal medicines are regulated much like pharmaceutical drugs are regulated in the US. There are over 160 herbal ingredients that are used in Kampō medicines. Some of these herbal medicines have been used clinically for various diseases as well as infectious diseases. The herbs are beneficial effects on fatigue, pain relief, reduction of diarrhoea, nausea, vomiting, protection of the liver, dispelling heat, cleaning toxins, and resolving swellings. The Japanese Kampō tradition uses fixed combinations of herbs in standardized proportions. The most widely prescribed Kampo medicine was kakkonto (70.2%), followed by daikenchuto (50.2%) and shakuyakukanzoto (49.2%). Figure 4.3 illustrates typical Japanese herbal medicines [9].

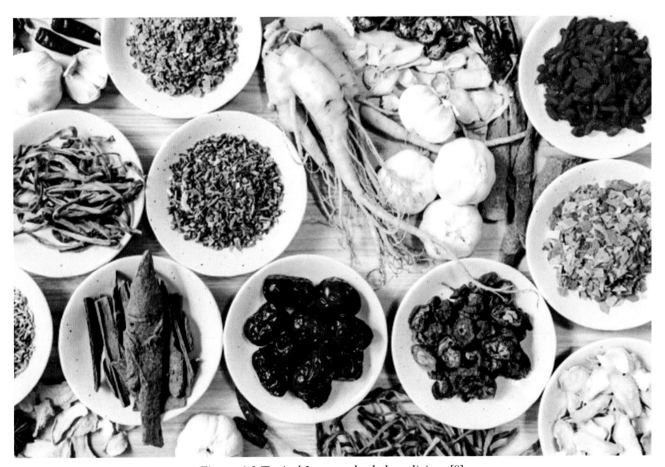

Figure 4.3 Typical Japanese herbal medicines [9].

The following herbs are typical traditional Japanese medicine readily available in Japanese markets [8,10,11]:

- *Yokukansan* was originally used to treat neurosis, insomnia, night crying, and irritability and/or agitation in infants. It is used globally for chronic migraine and headache.
- *Hochuekkito* is an influenza virus–preventing effect that has life-extending effectiveness and immunological responses.
- *Yokukansan* is a traditional Japanese herbal medicine that has been approved in Japan as a remedy for neurosis, insomnia, and irritability in children.
- *Bupleurum falcatum* is used as sai-ko (Bupleurum root), an antifebrile agent and to regulate liver functions.
- *O-ren:* Rhizome is a spice used to eliminate fever of the upper body, particularly in the heart.
- *Kakkonto* is a common Kampo that is designed to treat cold. It is made with a mixture of ginger, cinnamon, Chinese peony, licorice, jujube, and ephedra.
- *Benpiyaku* is found in medicine cabinet in every Japanese household. It is effective in regulating the movement of the large intestine, promoting bowel movement that is close to natural.
- *Kamiyoshosan* is popular Kampo medicine for menopause. It is designed to help ease hot flashes, stiff shoulders, fatigue, emotional distress, insomnia resulting from menopause.
- *Ashitaba* leaves can cure several ailments like heartburn, stomach ulcer, high blood pressure, hay fever, gout, and constipation. As a result, the ashitaba plant play a significant role in Japanese traditional medicine. It is shown in Figure 4.4 [12].

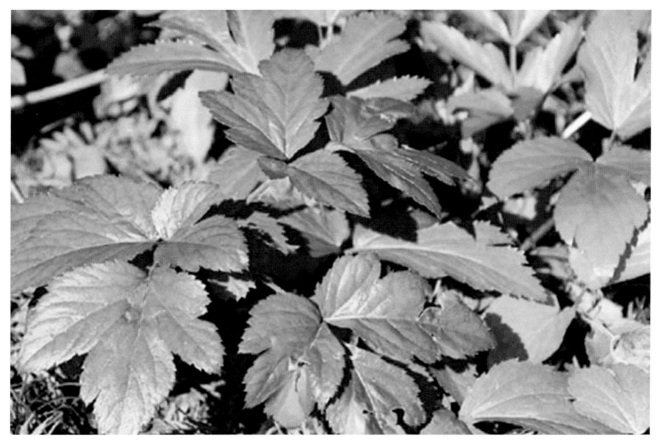

Figure 4.4 Ashitaba plant is significant in JTM [12].

- *Sho-saiko-to* is a basic Kampo prescription which has been shown to improve serum liver biochemistry levels in patients with chronic active hepatitis.
- *Boiogito* is a herbal medicine composed of six medicinal plants. It may also be a potent medication for preventing osteoarthritis.
- *Hochuekkito* is a traditional Japanese herbal medicine, which is composed of ten species of herbs. It has been used for the treatment of fatigue caused by common cold and severe weakness.

Some herbal herbs used in traditional Chinese medicine are also used in Japanese traditional medicine (JTM). Japanese herbal remedies sometimes contain powders that can be easily dissolved in warm water, in addition to capsules that are great for when you are on the go. These preparations are approved by the Japanese Food and Drug Administration. A factor that has strongly influenced the modern practice of Kampo was the formal recognition by the Japanese Ministry of Health.

4.6 APPLICATIONS OF JAPANESE TRADITIONAL MEDICINE

Kampo is a medical system that has been systematically organized based on the reactions of the human body to therapeutic interventions. It uses precisely measured herbs to treat illness, based on the skillful use of well-known formulas. Kampo has a holistic therapeutic approach because the mind and body are seen as one entity. Kampo medicines are usually prepared by blending natural herbs and boiling them in water to infuse them.

- *Treatment of Common Diseases:* Japanese Kampo medicines are a mixture of natural and herbal medicines that are available in Japan for the treatment of various diseases. They are often prescribed instead of, or alongside, allopathic medicines. Kampo medicines have proven to be effective for the treatment of a variety of inflammatory diseases, such as colitis, dermatitis, myocarditis, hepatitis, cardiomyopathy, and nephritis. Kampo is used for treating symptoms that are diagnosed as headaches, sense of fatigue, coldness, palpitation, stomach upset, constipation, diarrhea, dysmenorrhea, headache, and atopic dermatitis [13]. They have been used for various psychiatric disorders such as dementia, schizophrenia spectrum disorders, mood disorders, anxiety disorders, and personality disorders.
- *Virus Infection:* In Japan, some of these herbal medicines have been used to treat for various diseases as well as almost all infectious diseases. Traditional herbal medicines, Maoto and Hochuekkito, were clinically effective against influenza infectious disease [14].
- *Pain Relief:* An increasing number of Japanese patients complain of chronic pain for different reasons. These patients are often treated with Western drugs (such as opioid), all of which have side effects. Japanese traditional herbal medicine (Kampo) is widely used for pain management in outpatients with a lower incidence of side effects compared to Western medicine [15].
- *Frailty:* This is a state of increased vulnerability to poor resolution of homeostasis following stress, which increases the risk of adverse outcomes such as falls, delirium, and disability in the elderly. Frailty has recently gained considerable attention in terms of preventive care in Japan. The Japan Geriatrics Society defines frailty as a state of increased vulnerability in elderly people before the need for long-term care. At present, clinical studies are investigating Kampo medicines as frailty treatments. Researchers from Japan and China have recently collated 30 clinical studies detailing

Kampo's evidence on frailty. It is hoped that herbal medicines can become a mainstream treatment for frailty [16].

- *Acupuncture:* This is an age-old, Asian form of treatment that dates back more than 1,500 years. It is an important part of Japan's traditional medical practice and a significant part of their public health system. It involves inserting needles at specified points to help restore balance to the flow of Qi. The Japanese style of acupuncture is shown in Figure 4.5 [9].

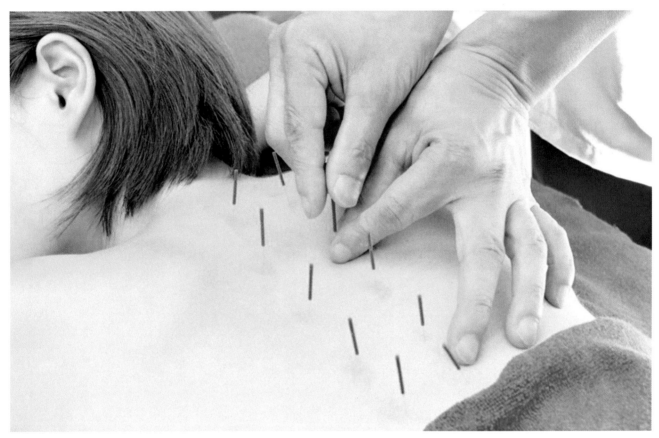

Figure 4.5 Japanese acupuncture [9].

Japanese acupuncture involves the shallow insertion of very fine needles using a guide tube to reduce pain and cause relaxation. Touching is emphasized in the pre-exam of Japanese acupuncture in order to determine proper needle insertion points and treatment strategy [17]. The ancient art of acupuncture in Japan continues to be practiced today by licensed practitioners. People turn to acupuncture to treat various ailments such as chronic pain, stress, digestive disorders, and infertility. Acupuncture is a drug-free treatment and is ideal for professional athletes. Japanese acupuncture is different from the Chinese style in the following respects [18]: (1) Palpation before the treatment, (2) Needle insertion methods, (3) Needle size, (4) Needle insertion depth, (5) Herbs as part of the acupuncture treatment, (6) Moxibustion, (7) Stronger sensation.

- *Massage Therapy*: Shiatsu is the most popular form of Japanese massage. In its original form, it uses the same topography of energy flow as things like Acupuncture, Qi gong, and moxibustion, but uses broad, flat hands to apply pressure as the primary actor. The word Shiatsu means "finger pressure" as it involves taking the healing energy from the practitioner and into the body of their patient [9]. Other types of massages include Anna massage, Ashiatsu massage, Nuru msaage, and Ampuku Hara abdominal massage.

- *Water Therapy:* Water is an indispensable constituent of life without which no life can exist in planet earth. More than 70% of planet earth is filled with water; around 60% of human body is made up of water. Traditional medicines across the world use water to treat various diseases. In Japan, water therapy employs water to treat various illness in human body. .Japanese water therapy is a holistic idea that suggests to take water in the empty stomach first in the morning and also take it in regular intervals. Water helps to keep your liver and kidney healthy. It also flushes the toxins. Figure 4.6 illustrates Japanese water therapy [19].

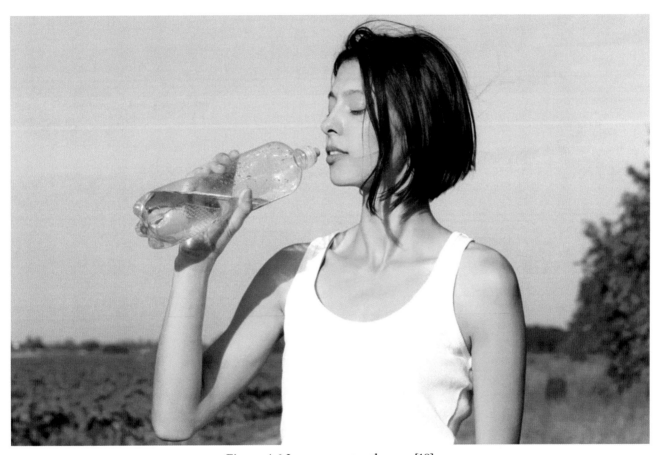

Figure 4.6 Japanese water therapy [19].

- *Ageing:* Ageing is major global concern. Japan has an ever-increasing aging population. We all desire to retain our youthfulness with radiant skin and without aging lines and wrinkles. With aging we are vulnerable to having physical issues and diseases. A good lifestyle and a certain kind of diet can help us keep younger for several years. The traditional products can help us to stay young for a longer period of time. The Japanese women have been known for retaining their youthfulness because of their unique diet plan and skin care. A herbal medicine known as Rikkunshito can help us to stay youthful and healthy. It can help maintain the youthfulness among the men and women across the globe. The herbal remedy is still under the experimental phase. A natural process of staying young is also possible. Eating less causes a delay in the ageing process and also delay in the arrival of age-related diseases and functional impairment [20].

- *Obesity:* The main cause of obesity includes genetic and environmental factors. Although drug therapy is available for obesity, it is highly risky. The Food and Drug Administration (FDA) only approved one antiobesity medication. Kampo medicine was not been recognized as a useful tool for the treatment of obesity until the 20th century [21].

- *Cancer:* An increasing number of patients with lung cancer are undergoing outpatient chemotherapy. Bone cancer pain control is difficult because it includes various characteristics of pain. Oral administration of Yokukansan (YKS) significantly alleviates cancer pain behavior. Radiotherapy is a standard treatment modality for patients with head and neck cancer. Oral mucositis induced by radiation or chemoradiation can cause devastating quality of life issues for patients undergoing treatment for head and neck cancer. In head and neck cancer patients undergoing chemoradiotherapy, oral ulcerative mucositis (OUM) is one of the most serious side effects. The traditional Japanese herbal medicine Hangeshashinto (HST) has beneficial effects for the treatment of oral ulcerative mucositis (OUM) in cancer patients

In Japan, Kampo is applied in almost all medical disciplines including psychiatry, hormone replacement therapy, Alzheimer's disease, coughing, diarrhea, nausea, eruption, anxiolytics, insomnia, hypertension, stroke, gastrointestinal disorders, weight loss, stiff shoulders, troubled skin, forgetfulness, stress, anxiety, and troubled stomach.

4.7 BENEFITS

Traditional Japanese medicine, Kampo, has repenetrated throughout Japanese society. It is used by over 80% of medical doctors in Japan because it produces fewer side effects. It serves as preventive medicine, an alternative to modern western medicine but also for daily healthcare and fitness regimens. Japanese life expectancy is at the top rank in the world.

Kampo is covered by national medical insurance. Prescription of Kampo medicine is limited to medical doctors. Prescription, manufacturing, and sale of Kampo are strictly regulated by the Japanese Ministry of Health, Labor and Welfare. The efficacy of traditional Japanese Kampo medicines for a number of conditions such as headache and pain has been reported. Modern medicine should consider the efficacy of traditional medicine as they may contain wisdom.

Other benefits of Kampo include [22].

- *Cost:* Kampo is relatively less expensive than Western medicine.
- *Lower Side Effects:* Kampo is beneficial in terms of a lower incidence of side effects compared to Western medicine.
- *Effective Treatment:* Japanese traditional herbal medicine is an effective and safe treatment. As a result, some physicians prescribe Kampo medicine to compensate for the shortcomings of modern medicine.
- *Customized Treatment:* Kampo is a tailor-made treatment. Patient preferences and patient expectation can play a role in complementary and alternative medicine trials. Japanese traditional herbal practitioners consider several factors such as age, international index of erectile function,

testosterone levels, etc. The efficacy and safety of Japanese traditional herbal medicine are enhanced by appropriate selection in individual patients.

- *Holistic Treatment:* Western medicine focuses on the sick parts of the body to identify and remove the cause of a sickness. As powerful as western medicine is, it is not versatile enough to cure all types of diseases. In contrast, Kampo does not just focus on the condition of diseased parts but checks the condition of the entire body and mind. While allopathic medicine looks at ailments in isolation, traditional Japanese medicine uses a holistic view of the body to correct natural imbalance.

- *Integrative Medicine:* Around the world, modern healthcare systems increasingly encourages integrative healthcare modalities that incorporate ancient wisdom. Kampo medicine is integrative as it has been used by Western physicians in addition to conventional medicine. Due to its high quality and safety, Kampo has been integrated into modern medicine and there is no separate medical license for traditional medicine in Japan.

These benefits are illustrated in Figure 4.7.

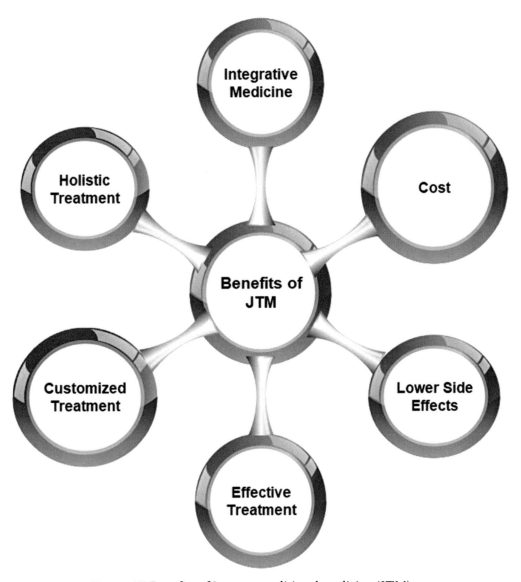

Figure 4.7 Benefits of Japanese traditional medicine (JTM).

4.8 CHALLENGES

Some skeptics doubt traditional medicine, based on the efficacy in clinical trials. Herbal medicines are still not fully accepted in clinical practice because researchers require more evidence regarding their appropriate and safe usage. Understanding that the only constant is change, Japanese modern practitioners continue to adapt to changes in medicine and social development. Researchers across the world are working on the efficacy of traditional medicine on chronic pain, chemotherapy-induced nausea, migraines, cancer, fibromyalgia, osteoarthritis, and alleviating labor pain [23].

Kampo formulations for prescription were approved based on experience. No clinical trials were conducted with dried extract prior to approval. There were no clear clinical data that showed its efficacy. Since Kampo is an individualized treatment, it is not suited for evaluations with statistical methodologies. With the era of evidence-based medicine in the 1990s, the Japan Society for Oriental Medicine (JSOM) established a special committee for evidence-based medicine in 2001 and began collecting high-grade clinical evidence for Kampo medicines [24]. The information on the interactions between herbal medicines and chemical drugs is necessary.

The World Health Organization took the initiative for globalization of traditional medicine since a large quantity of people in the world still depend on traditional medicine for healthcare. The acceptance of Kampo remedies into Japan's national health insurance system marked the start of the rapid growth of Kampo's market [25].

Other challenges include [26]:

- *Side Effects:* Due to the complexity of Kampo system, only an experienced practitioner can balance out medications in a way to avoid side effects.
- *Toxicity*: Some Kampo herbs are toxic. The toxic side effects can be minimized if prescribed and monitored by an experienced Kampo practitioner.
- *Mixing Western and Kampo Medicines:* Avoid mixing Western herbs with Kampo medications. Some patients have experienced kidney or liver problems after treatment with Kampo medications.
- *Lack of Regulation*: Within Japan, prescription, manufacture, and sale of Kampo is strictly regulated by the Japanese Ministry of Health, Labor and Welfare. Beyond Japan, Western Kampo practitioners practice as alternative healthcare providers in the United States. As such, they are largely unregulated.

4.9 TAKING KAMPO GLOBAL

The globalization of healthcare has not left traditional medicine behind. The World Health Organization (WHO) supports the integration of traditional medicine. Natural herbal products have attained their popularity as well in the recent times. Kampo, Japanese traditional medicine, has drawn attention around the world because it produces fewer adverse reactions. While the goal of Western medicine is to heal sickness itself, Kampo attempts to heal the person who is affected by the sickness. Researchers are urging more research on the Japanese herbal medicine, Kampo, as part of a push to increase awareness in global markets. Recent decades have seen a revival of Kampo medicine in medical practice within a context dominated by modern Western medicine. The development of modern ready-to-use drugs was directly related to the enormous increase in Kampo usage [27].

Kampo is primarily practiced in the West by acupuncturists, naturopaths, and Chinese medicine practitioners. Kampo medicine is taught in various universities including Takushoku University, Toyama Medical University, Iwate Medical University, and British School of Japanese Traditional Medicine. The Japan Liaison of Oriental Medicine (JLOM) is working toward the standardization of traditional medicine in the East Asia region in close coordination with the WHO.

4.10 CONCLUSION

The Japanese traditional medicine, Kampo, is a holistic and individualized treatment with a long tradition. It is getting more and more attention. Perhaps the most interesting aspect of Japanese medicine is the rapidity with which it became Westernized and scientific. Today, Kampō is integrated into the Japanese national health care system. Several graduate programs in Japanese traditional medicine can help one become a Kampo practitioner in this growing industry. Kampo medicine is now included in educational programs for medical students. For example, acupuncture and Integrative Medicine College in Berkeley, California focuses on teaching the Japanese style of acupuncture.

Japanese traditional herbal medicine can help you restore your natural balance. However, before choosing Kampo, you must do your homework by checking the qualifications of the Kampo practitioner and find out if it is the right treatment for you. Make sure you obtain Kampo medications from a trusted and reliable source. A good place to find a Kampo practitioner is with local Chinese herbalists or acupuncturists. More information about Japanese traditional medicine can be found in the books in [3,12,28-37] and the following related journals:

- *Journal of Herbal Medicine*
- *Journal of Ethnopharmacology.*
- *Chinese Journal of Integrative Medicine*
- *Journal of Integrative Medicine*
- *Journal of Alternative and Complementary Medicine*
- *Journal of Traditional and Complementary Medicine*
- *Advances in Traditional Medicine*
- *Traditional Medicine and Modern Medicine*
- *Alternative and Complementary Therapies*
- *Evidence-Based Complementary & Alternative Medicine*

REFERENCES

[1]   M. N. O. Sadiku, O. D. Olaleye, A. Ajayi-Majebi, and S. M. Musa, "Essence of Japanese Traditional Medicine," *International Journal of Trend in Research and Development*, vol. 8, no. 5, November-December 2021, pp. 322-326.

[2]   "The rise of 'made-in-Japan' Chinese herbal remedies," January 2018, https://asia.nikkei.com/Business/Business-trends/The-rise-of-made-in-Japan-Chinese-herbal-remedies

[3]   S. Dharmananda, *KAMPO MEDICINE: The Practice of Chinese Herbal Medicine in Japan.* ITM 2002.

[4] "What is Kampo,"
https://kampo-promotion.jp/en/what.html

[5] "What is Kampo ?" Kampo virtual class
https://www.keio-kampo.jp/vc/education1_1.html#:~:text=What%20is%20Kampo%3F,by%20 75%25%20of%20Japanese%20physicians

[6] K. Ogura et al., " Maoto, a traditional Japanese medicine, controls acute systemic inflammation induced by polyI:C administration through noradrenergic function," *Gene,* vol. 806, 2022.

[7] K. Watanabe et al., "Traditional Japanese Kampo medicine: Clinical research between modernity and traditional medicine—the state of research and methodological suggestions for the future," *Evidence-Based Complementary and Alternative Medicine*, February, 2011.

[8] T. Hatano, "Herbal drugs in traditional Japanese medicine," *Open Access,* Chapter 3, December 2012.

[9] "Top 4 Alternative/traditional Japanese medicine and therapy,"
https://www.metroresidences.com/jp-en/expat-life/japan/alternative-traditional-japanese-medicine-therapy/

[10] M. Matsumiya et al., "Japanese herbal medicine hochuekkito inhibits the expression of proinflammatory biomarker, inducible nitric oxide synthase, in hepatocytes," *Medicinal Chemistry,* vol. 2, no. 2, 2012, pp. 041-047.

[11] "Japanese medicine and medicated products,"
https://www.takaski.com/japanese-medicine-and-medicated-products/

[12] "Boost cellular health and prevent aging with this Japanese plant,"
https://yogaesoteric.net/en/boost-cellular-health-and-prevent-aging-with-this-japanese-plant/

[13] S. Arumugam and K. Watanabe, *Japanese Kampo Medicines for the Treatment of Common Diseases.* Elsevier, 2021.

[14] "A Kampo (traditional Japanese herbal) medicine, hochuekkito, pretreatment in mice prevented influenza virus replication accompanied with GM-CSF expression and increase in several defensin mRNA Levels," *Pharmacology*, vol. 91, 2013, pp. 314-321.

[15] M. Oohata et al., "Japanese traditional herbal medicine reduces use of pregabalin and opioids for pain in patients with lumbar spinal canal stenosis: a retrospective cohort study," *JA Clinical Reports,* vol. 3, 2017.

[16] G. Y. Lim, "Taking Kampo global: Researchers call for continued research into Japanese herbal medicine and frailty," May 2020,
https://www.nutraingredients.com/Article/2020/05/26/Taking-Kampo-global-Researchers-call-for-continued-research-into-Japanese-herbal-medicine-and-frailty?utm_source=copyright&utm_medium=OnSite&utm_campaign=copyright

[17] P. T. Chong, A. Greer,and S. Olkeriil, "Japanese medicine,"
https://slideplayer.com/slide/4847951/

[18] "A brief history of Japanese acupuncture & how it's different from Chinese acupuncture," January 2018,
https://www.aimc.edu/2018/01/16/a-brief-history-of-japanese-acupuncture-how-its-different-from-chinese-acupuncture/#:~:text=They%20were%20developed%20in%20Japan,much%20 more%20than%20Japanese%20acupuncture.&text=Japanese%20needles%20tend%20to%20 be,being%20sharper%20than%20Chinese%20needles.&text=Chinese%20needling%20fosters%20 more%20depth%20of%20insertion.

[19]   J. Aruchami, "Benefits of Japanese water therapy," September 2020,
https://discover.hubpages.com/health/Water-in-traditional-medicine

[20]   A. Khatoon, "Japanese traditional herbal medicine can help with a prolonged life span," February 2016,
https://trendingposts.net/trending-health-news/japanese-traditional-herbal-medicine-can-help-with-a-prolonged-life-span/

[21]   J. Yamakawa et al., "Significance of Kampo, Japanese traditional medicine, in the treatment of obesity: Basic and clinical evidence," *Evidence-Based Complementary and Alternative Medicine*, 2013.

[22]   I. Arai, "Clinical studies of traditional Japanese herbal medicines (Kampo): Need for evidence by the modern scientific methodology," *Integrative Medicine Research*, vol. 10, no.3, September 2021.

[23]   "Kampo: Japanese herbal medicine," Unknown Source.

[24]   I. Arai, "Clinical studies of traditional Japanese herbal medicines (Kampo): Need for evidence by the modern scientific methodology," *Integrative Medicine Research*, vol.10, no. 3, September 2021.

[25]   S. Yakubo ewt al., "Pattern classification in Kampo medicine," *Evidence-Based Complementary and Alternative Medicine*, 2014.

[26]   "KAMPO: Japanese herbal medicine," May 2016,
https://institutoflash786.org/2016/05/01/kampo-japanese-herbal-medicine/

[27]   K. Watanabe, "Traditional Japanese Kampo medicine: Clinical research between modernity and traditional medicine—the state of research and methodological suggestions for the future," *Evidence-Based Complementary and Alternative Medicine*, February 2011.

[28]   K. Otsuka, *Kampo, A Clinical Guide to Theory and Practice*. Singing Dragon, 2nd edition, 2016.

[29]   M. M. Lock, *East Asian Medicine in Urban Japan: Varieties of Medical Experience (Volume 3) (Comparative Studies of Health Systems and Medical Care)*. University of California Press, volume 3,1980.

[30]   A. Tsumura, *Kampo: How the Japanese Updated Traditional Herbal Medicine*. Japan Publications, 1991.

[31]   Y. Nobuo, *Western Medicine a Cure Full of Mistakes: Important Things Taught By Japanese Traditional Medicine Doctor Ayukawa Shizuka (Japanese Edition)*. Kindle Edition, 2020.

[32]   N. Dawes, *Fukushin and Kampo: Abdominal Diagnosis in Traditional Japanese and Chinese Medicine*. Kindle Edition, 2020.

[33]   K. Triplett, *Buddhism and Medicine in Japan*. De Gruyter, 2019.

[34]   N. Dawes, K. Watanabe, and K. Ossenfort, *Fukushin and Kampo : Abdominal Diagnosis in Traditional Japanese and Chinese Medicine*. Singing Dragos (US), 2020.

[35]   Society of Traditional Japanese Medicine Staff, *Traditional Japanese Acupuncture : Fundamentals of Meridian Therapy*. Complementary Medicine Press, 2003.

[36]   J. Belleme, Japanese Foods That Heal : Using Traditional Japanese Ingredients to Promote Health, Longevity and Well-Being. Tuttle Publishing, 2007.

[37]   R. Rister, *Japanese Herbal Medicine: The Healing Art of Kampo*. Avery, 1999.

5

European Traditional Medicine

"Prevention is always better than cure!" – Common saying

5.1 INTRODUCTION

Throughout written history, medicine and agriculture have guided the study of plants, animals, microorganisms, and marine organisms in order to alleviate and treat diseases. The development of new drugs by pharmaceutical companies relying purely on modern technology appears to be reaching its limit. Increasing attention has been paid recently to natural products [1],

Traditional medicine (TM) (or folk medicine) is a term that usually refers to medical systems such as traditional Chinese medicine and Indian medicine. It refers to practices, approaches, knowledge, and cultural beliefs not based on scientific evidence that are applied to treat, diagnose, and prevent illness. The World Health Organization (WHO) provided a definition of TM as "the sum total of knowledge, skills and practices based on the theories, beliefs and experiences of different cultures that are used to maintain health, as well as to prevent, diagnose, improve or treat physical and mental illness." TM is also known as herbal medicine, natural medicine, phytomedicine, and botanical medicine [2].

TM is regarded "complementary," "alternative" or "non-conventional" medicine. Herbal and traditional medicinal products are being used for healthcare all over the world. TM is the oldest form of medicine in the world. In ancient time, people believed the diseases were caused by spirits and sin. Although traditional medicine is important due to its long history, it is often underestimated health resource. According to the WHO, more than 70 % of the world population is currently treated with traditional medicines. A large fraction of the population in many developing countries rely on traditional medicine to meet healthcare needs. Although modern medicine may exist side-by-side with such traditional medicine, TMs have often maintained their popularity for historical and cultural reasons [3].

Traditional medicines have been a part of human history all over the world, with knowledge being transferred from generation to generation. In recent years, advances in the Western medical have led much of the knowledge of traditional medicines of our ancestors to be forgotten. Traditional healing is culturally sensitive in nature and takes into account the cultural and historical backgrounds of patients [4].

Europe has been using traditional medicines for over hundreds or even thousands of years. European traditional medicine (ETM) essentially refers to traditional therapies that have their origin in Europe and is practiced throughout the European Union (EU).

It consists of various approaches of traditional medical healing systems in Europe, beginning with Hippocrates in ancient Greece and ending in current times. It primarily deals with local plants and their medicinal benefits. Today these alternative approaches to medicine have gained a lot in popularity with patients. In spite of this popularity, there is little dialog between allopathic practitioners and ETM users.

This chapter provides an introduction on European traditional medicine (ETM). It begins by providing a brief historical background on ETM. It discusses the concept of ETM and its herbal medicines. It provides some applications of ETM and its globalization. It highlights the benefits and challenges of ETM. The last section concludes with comments.

5.2 BRIEF HISTORY OF ETM

Europe's landscape has been shaped by centuries of diverse farming and forestry traditions. Europe has shared a vibrant history in the use of herbal medicines since ancient times. Written history allows tracing back European medical traditions to Greek antiquity. The basis of European medicine was laid down during Greek antiquity and the period of the Roman Empire. The most eminent and influential classic author was Hippocrates of Kos, who successfully combined both botanical and medical skills. Hippocrates is acknowledged as a father of western medicine. The Arabs translated Greek medical knowledge into Arabic. The European medical tradition was continuously updating terminologies and adding new names, novel pathologies, and interpreting previous texts in contemporaneous term [5].

The first historic trend toward the globalization of traditional medicines was linked to the trade along important terrestrial or sea routes during the Middle Ages. In 2004, the European Parliament adopted "traditional use" for an herbal substance as a basis for using it as a safe product for treating a specified medical conditions. In 2007, there was the first international Congress to discuss together ethnomedicine of European Countries in search of clinical evidence.

In May 2011, it is now forbidden to sell traditional herbal medicinal products in the European Union without the necessary registration. Entire medicinal traditions like the Indian Ayurveda and Chinese traditional medicine are excluded from registration because they have not been officially used in Europe for 15 to 30 years. Consequently, very few of those medicinal herbs have been registered during the transition period from 2004 to now. This caused herbal practitioners and healers from India and China to complain most bitterly from being unceremoniously pushed out of Europe [6].

European traditional medicine is currently in a state of decline. The traditional knowledge about ETM treatment eroded by the deep economical and social changes of the past few decades.

5.3 CONCEPT OF EUROPEAN TRADITIONAL MEDICINE

Traditional medicine is based on medical knowledge developed by indigenous cultures that incorporates plants, animals, and spiritual therapies designed to treat illness or disease. In Europe, there is a very long history of traditional medicine, which many European citizens still rely and trust in it for treating minor and sometimes severe diseases. Traditional European medicine (TEM) includes traditional therapies that have their origin in Europe. TEM has been used traditionally for health purposed in all European nations [7].

The original intent of European legislation on traditional medicinal products was to offer an option for products with substantial medical use in Europe. The legislation was designed to put a high barrier for herbal medicine registration and to make sure they would be no threat to conventional, pharmaceutical medicines. Through legislation, the European Union (EU) has harmonized legislation on herbal and traditional medicinal products. The harmonization is meant to facilitate access to the market in different member states and to guarantee safety in appropriate application of traditional herbal medicinal products. EU assesses the quality, effectiveness, and safety of traditional herbal medicinal products before they have access to the market. The quality of traditional medicine products varies enormously. The quality must meet the same criteria as any other medicinal products [8]. The safety of TM products is a top concern for their transition into mainstream use. To prove its effectiveness, TM must go through rigorous laboratory testing just like modern drugs. There are some dangerous herbs that bypass scrutiny by the general public because of their supposed healing properties. Starting from April of 2011, if an herbal medicinal product has not received full marketing authorization, it will be taken off the shelves of pharmacies. Figure 5.1 shows a garden full of herbs at Hollersbach [9].

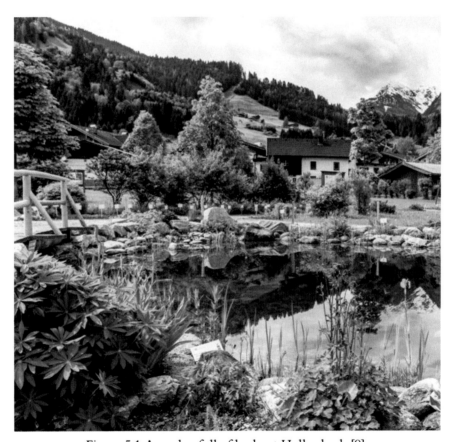

Figure 5.1 A garden full of herbs at Hollersbach [9].

In Europe, there are two ways for authorizing medicinal products: a centralized and a mutual recognition procedure. A number of international organizations are responsible for controlling medicines. These include the European Medicines Agency, the World Health Organization, the United Nations Office on Drugs and Crime, and the International Narcotics Control Board. The European Union has passed 139,338 directives, regulations, and decisions since 1980.

Important key institutions for ETM are the European Directorate for the Quality of Medicines & HealthCare (EDQM), the European Medicines Agency (EMA), and The European Herbal and Traditional medicine Practitioners Association (EHTPA).

- *EDQM:* The EDQM is located in Strasbourg, France. It supports the implementation and monitoring of the application of quality standards on medicinal products. It also provides reference standards for assays and tests.
- *EMA:* This is a decentralized agency of the European Union located in Amsterdam, the Netherlands. Its main objective is to coordinate the network of competent national authorities on medicinal products within the EU. It is responsible for the scientific evaluation of medicines for use in the EU. The Committee on Herbal Medicinal Products (HMPC) is the scientific committee within EMA, and is responsible for establishing EU herbal monographs, which address the efficacy and safety of herbal substances.
- *EHTPA:* This was founded in 1993 when it was clear that the practice of TM in Europe might undergo a radical change. It is an umbrella organization representing professional associations of herbal/traditional medicine practitioners offering European herbal medicine, Chinese herbal medicine, Ayurveda, and traditional Tibetan medicine. EHTPA is committed to developing herbal/traditional medicine and enhancing the legal basis of practice across EU Member states.

5.4 EUROPEAN HERBAL MEDICINES

Herbal medicine is the therapeutic use of plants to treat disease and enhance wellbeing. Western herbal medicine practice is based on European herbal medicines. The main aim of herbal medicine is to return the body to a state of natural balance, so that it can start healing itself. The demand for natural plant-based remedies is constantly increasing.

Traditional medicines are made using different parts of the plant like roots, tubers, barks, flowers, stems, seeds, berries, leaves, even whole plants and herbs. Many traditional medicines are made by crushing leaves, resulting in a mixture. A medicinal plant can be regarded as a food, a dietary supplement or a herbal medicine. Spices and herbs are an important ingredient in many traditional medical approaches. Herbs are essentially foods provided by God to feed, nourish, heal, cleanse, and renew our bodies

The European Union takes a somewhat cautious approach to herbal medicines. The European framework has provided a powerful regulation model for harmonization of scientific assessment and facilitation of product marketing. The European regulatory framework provides definitions for herbal medicinal products, traditional herbal medicinal products, herbal substances, and herbal preparations [10]:

- *Herbal medicinal products:* Any medicinal product exclusively containing as active ingredients one or more herbal substances in combination with one or more such herbal preparations.
- *Traditional herbal medicinal products:* An herbal medicinal product that fulfils the conditions laid down in Article 16a(1) of Directive 2001/83/EC. Vitamins and minerals may be added if their action is ancillary to the herbal constituent(s).

- *Herbal substances:* Herbal substances are precisely defined by the plant part used and the botanical name according to the binomial system.
- *Herbal preparations:* Preparations obtained by subjecting herbal substances to treatments such as extraction, distillation, expression, fractionation, purification, concentration, or fermentation.

Popular traditional European medicine or home remedies include:

- *Dictamnus:* This is a complex of different species. It was a popular name for a group of medicinal herbaceous plant species, which since the 4th century have been used for gynaecological problems and other illnesses.
- *Peucedanum Ostruthium:* This grows mainly at altitudes above 1200 m and is native to the Alpine region of Bavaria. Essential oil, tannins, and coumarins are the main active substances.
- *Mushrooms:* This is macroscopic fungi. Mushrooms from traditional European medicine have the potential to be used in modern medicine.
- *Lemon balm, camomile, mallow and calendula,* combined as a tea, settles the stomach.

Traditional medicines are used for treatment and prevention of various diseases or illness. Figure 5.2 shows some traditional medicines [11].

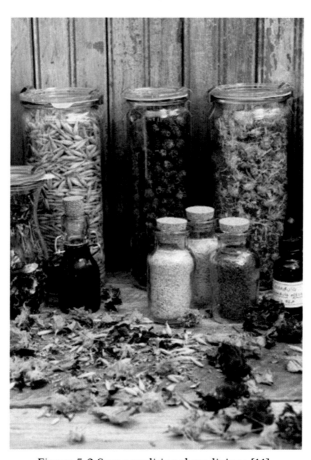

Figure 5.2 Some traditional medicines [11].

Figure 5.3 illustrates various uses of traditional European medicine. The basic approach in the EU is to assess the quality, efficacy, and safety of traditional herbal medicinal products before they get access to the market.

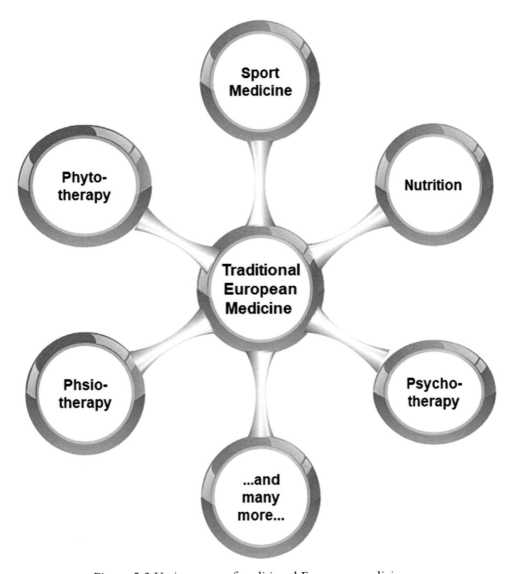

Figure 5.3 Various uses of traditional European medicine.

5.5 APPLICATIONS OF ETM

Herbal medicine is essential for targeting root causes of disease. There is a global and growing interest in the integration of herbal and traditional medicines. The European traditional herbal medicinal products can treat the following health issues.

- *Ear Acupuncture:* Auricular acupuncture is a diagnostic and treatment system based on normalizing the body's dysfunction through stimulation of points on the ear. It is an acupuncture technique similar to reflexology and is speculated that the technique works. Thus stimulation of a reflex point in the ear can relieve symptoms of distant pathology with a reliable duration. One problem with auricular acupuncture is that there are so many maps of the ear and little agreement exists regarding point location [13].
- *Alzheimer's Disease:* This is currently estimated to be the most abundant aging-related neurodegenerative disorder worldwide. It is today diagnosed based on the extent and type of

memory loss in patients. Plants used in the European traditional medicine is used to address multiple of Alzheimer's disease, until the molecular origin of the disease is unraveled [14].

- *Women's Healthcare*: Women experience unique conditions such as the menstrual cycles, pregnancy, childbirth, and breastfeeding that can adversely affect their health status, quality of life, social integration, and access to education. Herbal drugs have been used as additional or alternative treatments to conventional drugs to treat women's health problems, such as menstrual disorders, infertility, and dysfunctions of pregnancy, labor, urogenital diseases, and menopause [15].
- *Other Diseases:* Other health problems that ETM can heal include [10, 16]:
  - ➤ Skin disease, including eczema, psoriasis, acne, acne rosacea, urticaria
  - ➤ Gastrointestinal disorders, including acid indigestion, irritable bowel syndrome, chronic constipation, inflammatory bowel disease
  - ➤ Gynaecological conditions, including premenstrual syndrome and dysmenorrhoea, endometriosis, infertility
  - ➤ Chronic fatigue syndrome
  - ➤ Respiratory conditions, including asthma, bronchitis, and chronic coughs, rhinitis, and sinusitis
  - ➤ Arthritic conditions (e.g. osteoarthritis, gout and rheumatoid arthritis)
  - ➤ Urinary conditions including chronic cystitis, urinary tract infections, kidney stones
  - ➤ Psychological problems (e.g. depression, anxiety)
  - ➤ Cough and cold
  - ➤ Sleep disorders and temporary insomnia
  - ➤ Skin disorders and minor wounds
  - ➤ Loss of appetite

5.6 GLOBALIZATION OF ETM

Across the globe, top research bodies, medical practitioners, policymakers, and pharmaceutical companies are working together to bring traditional medicine into the twenty first century. They are serious about integrating traditional medicine into modern healthcare. Many nations are working actively to harness and regulate TM. Efforts to make traditional medicines mainstream have to cope with varying regulation. Every nation follows different regulatory policies. Much still needs to be done before a global standard for TM is agreed. Loose regulation means there are as many fake remedies and false practitioners as genuine treatments and practitioners. It is often difficult to distinguish between traditional treatments backed by research and those with unproven claims.

Due to the participation of many companies, the global market for herbal medicines is highly fragmented. A number of regional businesses are producing herbal products and the increasing technological advancements in the herbal medicines sector are accelerating the market competitiveness. Notable players of the market include Arkopharma, Bayer AG, BEOVITA, Hishimo Pharmaceuticals, Schaper & Brümmer, Venus Pharma GmbH, Dasherb Corp., Arizona Natural Products, Blackmores, and Himalaya Global Holdings Ltd. [17].

Globalization of traditional medicines is an ongoing process. It allows interactions between European traditional medicines and those from Asia, such as traditional Chinese medicine (TCM). Globalization is affecting the market within the EU. European herbal medicinal products have been exported worldwide, while traditional medicines from other parts of the world have been imported to the EU. Due to globalization, the Committee on Herbal Medicinal Products (HMPC) have been motivated to include issues related to non-European traditional medicines (such as Chinese herbal medicines) into the work program [18]. Traditional medicine has much to offer global health. This will require collaboration between developed and developing nations.

5.7 BENEFITS

Traditional medicines are becoming popular with patients. They are increasingly considered for prevention and treatment of the novel coronavirus, COVID-19. The prime beneficiaries of TM are the large European phytopharmaceutical companies. Only a very small portion of the total number of medicinal herbs get through the EU door [10]. TEM, however, is most often used as a synonym for the local herbal medicine.

Healthcare professionals with an education in traditional medicine can provide prescriptions for individuals. Global regulatory frameworks on herbal medicines and traditional medicines have been developed. The regulation of herbal and traditional medicines doubtless has the overall objective of safeguarding public health.

Other benefits include:

- *New Remedy:* Traditional medicines provide alternation solutions to modern medicine, which cannot cure all diseases. Modern medicine is desperately short of new treatments. Drugs take years to get through research, development, and commercialization, at enormous cost. So scientists and pharmaceutical companies are increasingly searching TM for new drug sources.
- *Safety and Efficacy:* Herbal products have been used since ancient time. There is expertise and experience in using and preparing them. Safety awareness concerning them have developed on the basis of longtime experience and through the help of science.
- *Holistic Treatment:* This refers the treatment of the complete person, physically, psychologically, socially, and spiritually in the prevention and management of disease. A holistic approach implies that the care provider finds out a patient's whole life situation. Nutrition, homeopathy, exercise, prayer, meditation and acupuncture are other treatments that may be used together with conventional medicine as part of a holistic approach. Traditional and holistic medicine may include acupuncture, Ayurveda, Yoga, homeopathy, homeopathy, and naturopathy.

5.8 CHALLENGES

There is no globally accepted set of definitions of traditional medicine. It is often difficult to apply modern standardized tests to TM products. Efforts to make traditional medicines mainstream will need to cope with regulations locally and globally. TM is often used with conventional medicines, making potential pharmacokinetic interactions a cause for concern. While European government must ensure the adequate availability of essential traditional medicines, it must introduce measures to reduce the possibility of their being used inappropriately.

Other challenges include [8,19,20]:

- *Safety:* The safety of some TMs has been recently called into question. The greatest challenge in traditional medicine was the need for more technical guidance on research and evaluation relating to the safety, efficacy, and quality of treatments. Efforts to incorporate TM into modern healthcare and ensure that it meets safety and efficacy requirements are far from complete.
- *Bad Reputation:* Although several people are looking for a viable alternative to "western medicine," sensationalism, fear mongering, and some scandals have damaged the reputation of the traditional medicine. There will be many fake remedies and false practitioners. It is always difficult to distinguish between fake and genuine traditional treatments.
- *Quality:* This is an essential requirement to guarantee wise usage of any medicinal product. Quality is already defined at the level of the starting material
- *Endangered Species:* The increasing demand for the ingredients for traditional medicines is endangering some plants and animals. In Kenya for example, local medicinal use are almost exclusively harvested from the wild, and much more material is used than previously thought.
- *Variable Dosage:* Dosage of TM is varied. Modern medicine demands dosages that are standardized based on factors such as bodyweight or disease severity. Traditional healers are more likely to give patients a unique dosage or combination of medicines that is decided during the consultation.
- *Toxicity:* Herbal products are toxic, unnatural man-made substances. They need to be proven safe before unleashing them on the public.
- *Intellectual Property Rights:* A striking difference between traditional and modern medicines is the legal protection of knowledge. Knowledge about TM was passed on and written down from generation to generation. Protecting intellectual property (IP) rights of traditional medicines, which are a form of cultural expression, is a thorny issue.
- *Culture Clash:* This is the issue of combining traditional medicines and modern drugs. The belief system that accompanies traditional medicine can sometimes interfere with modern treatments. If a traditional medicine is considered clinically ineffective by modern standards, it does not mean it cannot work as a therapy.
- *Integration:* Researchers around the world are concerned about integrating traditional medicine into modern healthcare. However, traditional medicines require reassessment before being integrated into mainstream medicine. Integrating traditional and modern medicines faces some challenges due to the key differences in how traditional and modern medicines are practiced, evaluated, and managed.
- *No Regulations:* The regulation of traditional medicines has the main objective of safeguarding public health. With loose or no regulations, anyone who calls himself an herbalist can prepare traditional medicines on their own premises and practice them on patients. A harmonized regulatory approach applying a unique best practice and mutual acceptance around the world is an uphill task. However, there are already regional regulatory networks established on different continents, such as Europe, Asia, and South America. The WHO is developing international guidelines and technical standards to help nations control traditional medicines. International communication and cooperation within the scientific community and regulators are needed to develop unified regulatory policies for herbal and traditional medicines to thrive.
- *Non-medical Use:* Non-medical use of over-the-counter medicines has become an increasing concern in Europe. Some people who have no medical reasons for using medicines use them for

recreational or enhancement purposes. The non-medical use of medicines in combination with other drugs or medicines can lead to interactions that may increase harms or result in death.

• *Medicine over Internet:* The increasing availability of medicines over the Internet poses a major challenge that will require the development of new policies. Many of these will involve law enforcement rather than health and social responses. A clearer understanding of the sources of the medicines appearing on different markets will be crucial for success here.

• *Non-European Herbs:* The current EU legislation requires 15-year minimum medicinal use period in the EU. This is a major obstacle to the registration of non-European traditional herbal medicinal products. The registration mandated by the EU does not regard all herbs but only those herbs that are sold as medicines.

• *Globalization:* A company must willing to handle some challenges if it wants to apply for access to the global market. Drug manufacturing companies face great challenges when trying to gain access to different markets for traditional medicines. They must follow different legislations, requirements, and standards. They are compelled to develop different dossiers to different national authorities.

Some of these challenges are displayed in Figure 5.5.

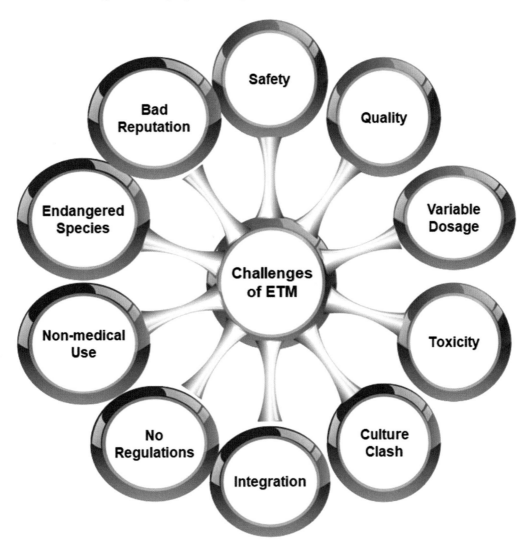

Figure 5.5 Challenges of European traditional medicine (ETM).

5.9 CONCLUSION

The knowledge of traditional medicine is increasingly drawing attention worldwide due to its significant role in meeting the global public health needs. There is a global and growing interest in the integration of herbal and traditional medicines.

Research into traditional medicines remains controversial. The scientific community should increase their knowledge about traditional medicine. Nearly 40 nations now provide high-level education and training programs on traditional medicine. National governments and local communities should encourage the development of the traditional medicines. They should establish systems for the testing of TM and for qualifying and licensing TM practitioners. A good documentation of traditional medicinal knowledge may also improve the use of TM and promote its commercialization [9].

Europe is a leader in herbal medicine. Herbs are naturally occurring plant products with recognized potential effects, intended to supplement drugs. They used mostly as nutrition supplements. Those who are sick about Big Pharm controlling everything can use alternative remedies. Educated use and quality control are required for using TM [21]. Today, courses of traditional medicines are offered online [11]. There is the University of Traditional Medicine located in the city of Yerevan, Armenia where students from different nationalities learn about traditional medicine [22]. The university is shown in Figure 5.4 [23]. More information about European traditional medicine can be found in the books in [24-27] and the following related journals:

- *Journal of Herbal Medicine*
- *Journal of Ethnopharmacology*
- *European Journal of Herbal Medicine*
- *European Journal of Integrative Medicine*
- *The Traditional Home Doctor (European Medical Journal)*

REFERENCES

[1] H. Yuan et al., "The traditional medicine and modern medicine from natural products," *Molecules,* vol. 21, 2016.

[2] A. Hossaini, B. Talukder, and A. Inban, "A history of traditional usage, efficacy and prospect of plant-derived medicine," *European Academic Research,* vol 8, no. 7, October 2020, pp. 4293-4302.

[3] M. N. O. Sadiku, O. D. Olaleye, A. Ajayi-Majebi, and S. M. Musa, "European traditional medicine," *International Journal of Trend in Research and Development,* vol. 8, no. 5, November-December 2021, pp. 307-309.

[4] A. Pieroni et al., "The European heritage of folk medicines and medicinal foods: Its contribution to the CAMs of tomorrow," *Evidenced-Based Complementary Alternative Medicine,* vol. 2013, April 2013.

[5] M. Leonti1 and R. Verpoorte, "Traditional Mediterranean and European herbal medicines," *Journal of Ethnopharmacology,* vol. 199, March 2017, pp.161-167.

[6] "Herbal medicines in Europe - Italy shows way out of impasse," July 2011, http://www.laleva.org/eng/2011/07/herbal_medicines_in_europe_-_italy_shows_way_out_of_impasse.html

[7] W. Peschel, "The traditional herbal medicine directive within the European regulatory framework for herbal products," *Boletín Latinoamericano y del Caribe de Plantas Medicinales y Aromáticas,* vol. 6, no.4, 2007, pp. 102 – 111.

[8] "Traditional medicine for modern times: Facts and figures," June 2015, https://www.scidev.net/global/features/traditional-medicine-modern-times-facts-figures/

[9] "Traditional European healing," https://www.salzburgerland.com/en/traditional-european-healing/

[10] W. Knoess and J. Wiesner, "The globalization of traditional medicines: Perspectives related to the European union regulatory environment," *Engineering,* vol.5, no. 1, 2019, pp. 22-31.

[11] "Online herbal medicine making course outline," https://chestnutherbs.com/online-herbal-classes/herbal-medicine-making-course/

[13] L. Gori and F. Firenzuoli, "Ear acupuncture in European traditional medicine," *Evidence-Based Complementary and Alternative Medicine,* vol. 4, suppl. 1, September 2007, pp. 13-16.

[14] E. S. B. Lobbens et al., "Screening of plants used in the European traditional medicine to treat memory disorders for acetylcholinesterase inhibitory activity and anti amyloidogenic activity," *Journal of Ethnopharmacology,* vol.200, March 2017, pp. 66-73.

[15] R. Motti et al., "Traditional herbal remedies used in women's health care in Italy: A review," *Human Ecology,* vol. 47, 2019, pp. 941–972.

[16] "What can herbal medicine help you with?" https://www.bewelldevon.co.uk/herbal-medicine/

[17] "Herbal medicine market trends, size estimation, regional insights, future growth, sales projection and industry overview by 2027," December 2021, https://www.medgadget.com/2021/12/herbal-medicine-market-trends-size-estimation-regional-insights-future-growth-sales-projection-and-industry-overview-by-2027.html

[18] R. Abbott, "Documenting traditional medical knowledge," March 2014, https://www.wipo.int/export/sites/www/tk/en/resources/pdf/medical_tk.pdf

[19] European Monitoring Centre for Drugs and Drug Addiction, "Non-medical use of medicines: Health and social responses," 2021, https://www.emcdda.europa.eu/publications/mini-guides/non-medical-use-of-medicines-health-and-social-responses_en

[20] "Integrating modern and traditional medicine: Facts and figures," May 2010, https://www.scidev.net/global/features/integrating-modern-and-traditional-medicine-facts-and-figures/

[21] "Dark times for herbal medicine in Europe," March 2011, https://anh-usa.org/dark-times-for-herbal-medicine-in-europe/

[22] "University of Traditional Medicine," https://www.eklavyaoverseas.com/university-of-traditional-medicine/

[23] "University of Traditional Medicine," https://www.studymedicineeurope.com/university-of-traditional-medicine

[24] I. V. Zevin, N. Altman, L. V. Zevin, *A Russian Herbal: Traditional Remedies for Health and Healing.* Healing Arts Press, 1997.

[25] C. Müller-Ebeling, C. Rätsch and W. D. Storl, *Witchcraft Medicine: Healing Arts, Shamanic Practices, and Forbidden Plants.* Inner Traditions, 2003.

[26] A. Chevallier, *Encyclopedia of Herbal Medicine: 550 Herbs and Remedies for Common Ailments.* DK, 3rd edition, 2016.

[27] K. Hostettmann et al. (eds.), *Phytochemistry of Plants Used in Traditional Medicine (Proceedings of the Phytochemical Society of Europe, 37).* Clarendon Press, 1995.

6

African Traditional Medicine

"Your food is supposed to be your medicine and your medicine is supposed to be your food." - African Proverb

6.1 INTRODUCTION

The desire to achieve good health cuts across national boundaries. Every region of the world has had one form of traditional medicine at some stage in its history. According to the World Health Organization (WHO), 80% of the emerging world's population relies on traditional medicine. Traditional medicine (TM) refers to health practices that incorporate plant, animal, and mineral to treat, diagnose, and prevent illnesses. It is basically a system of health practice that is based on indigenous knowledge.

Traditional medicine is variously known as ethno-medicine, folk medicine, native healing, complementary medicine or alternative medicine. An understanding of traditional medicine in any community should acknowledge its culture and history. Although TM has not been officially recognized in most countries, it remains a much neglected part of global healthcare due to many challenges it faces. In most developed nations, traditional medicine it is often described as "folk medicine" or "alternative medicine," offered as an alternative to conventional modern medicine [1].

Africa is the second largest continent in the world after Asia. It is the cradle of mankind with cultural diversity. African traditional medicine (ATM) is regarded as the oldest of all therapeutic systems. Traditional medicine is a major socio-economic and socio-cultural heritage for Africans with a long history of use. Before the advent of Western medicine, Africans had developed their own effective way of dealing with health issues. Traditional African medicine refers to indigenous forms of healing that are practiced all over the continent of Africa. It is the accumulation of knowledge and practices based on the cultural experiences used to maintain health as well as treat physical and mental illnesses. ATM is fundamentally different from modern medicine or other TMs such as Chinese traditional medicine and Indian traditional medicine [2,3].

This chapter provides an introduction on African traditional medicine. It begins by giving a brief history of ATM. It discusses the concept and components of ATM. It covers herbal medicine and traditional medicines from some selected African nations. It discusses regulation and applications of ATM. It compares traditional and modern medicines. It highlights the benefits and challenges of ATM. It addresses the effort to globalize ATM. The last section concludes with comments.

6.2 BRIEF HISTORY OF ATM

African traditional medicine is perhaps the oldest of all therapeutic systems. It has evolved over centuries. African history and culture began in ancient Egypt, which was the birthplace of world civilization. Egypt presided over a unified Black Africa until its ideas and technologies were stolen and its record of accomplishments obscured by Europeans. The arrival of the Europeans was a noticeable turning point in the history of African ancient culture.

Before colonialization, Africans had always believed in God and the ancestors and had been profoundly spiritual. As colonialism and Christianity spread through Africa, colonialists built general hospitals and Christian missionaries built private ones, with the hopes of making headway against widespread diseases. To some extent, colonialism, foreign religion, and Western education have negatively affected the perception of ATM. The European system of medicine was introduced by colonisers, while traditional medicine was outrightly banned. The period between 1840 and 1860 marked a significant innovation in tropical medicine. The invention of quinine was crucial to the treatment of malaria. From this point of view, the institutionalization of the modern healthcare system can be seen as one of the many "legacies" of Western encroachment in Africa [4].

In post independence Africa, concerted efforts have been made to recognize traditional medicine as important aspect of healthcare delivery system in Africa. Today, there is a concern for assessing and evaluating the effectiveness of the ATM across the world.

6.3 CONCEPT OF AFRICAN TRANDITIONAL MEDICINE

Keep in mind that Africa is a continent, comprising of 54 nations (such as Egypt, South Africa, Nigeria, Ghana, Kenya, etc.) each with its diverse traditional medicines. Different nations and ethnic groups have developed different healthcare systems and treatment strategies. In spite of these, profound similarities exist in the practice of traditional medicine in different African countries.

Traditional medicine in Africa is used extensively for cultural and economic reasons. African traditional medicine is the African indigenous system of healthcare. It is based on the culture that believes that good health indicates a correct relationship between people and their supernatural environment. It involves collecting, conserving, utilizing, and applying medicinal plants for the cure, prevention, and promotion of physical and spiritual well-being of the people. The traditional healer's ability to know the root cause of sickness and treat it is considered a gift from both God and the practitioner's ancestors. Traditional medical knowledge may be passed on orally from generation to generation or it may be taught in officially recognized universities.

The philosophy of African medical practice is rooted in the African world view, the African way of understanding the visible world. Some scholars have referred to this worldview as Afrocentricity. Afrocentricity is an approach to scholarship that encourages Africans to articulate their own system of values. It is a way of looking at life from "a black perspective" as opposed to what had been considered the "white perspective" [5]. The strongest philosophical argument for traditional medical practice is that it is holistic; it incorporates the personal, social, physical, and spiritual aspects of man. From African viewpoint, diseases are mostly caused by evil spirits, witchcraft/sorcery, gods, ancestors, or nature. Illness is considered as due to supernatural causes such as angered spirits, witchcraft, or evil spirits [6]. Africans believe that sickness and diseases are caused by evil spirits, gods or goddesses and they should be appeased and consulted to know what to do.

African traditional medicine is a holistic health practice that uses indigenous herbalism combined with some aspects of spirituality. It involves the direct application of herbal remedies, animal parts, or mineral materials for healing purposes. It is still the main source of healthcare delivery in almost all Africa nations in spite of the growth of religious enlightenment, Western civilization, and modern medicine. It is often regarded as an alternative or complementary system of medicine.

The traditional healer is one who provides healthcare using herbs, minerals, animal parts, incantations, exorcism, and other methods, based on the cultures and beliefs of his people. When an animal sacrifice is involved in the healing process, the slaughtering of an animal must be done properly and at an appropriate place. Blood is an important aspect in the traditional African religion and custom. The traditional healer typically diagnoses and treats the psychological basis of an illness before prescribing medicines. The primary healers in traditional African medicine are herbalists, diviners, and midwives. Herbalists use animal parts, plants/herbs and minerals to cure diseases. Diviners employ spiritual means to determine the root cause underlying any sickness or bad luck. Midwives use herbs and indigenous plants in aiding pregnancy and childbirth. Traditional African healers may employ counselling, charms, incantations, and casting of spells [7].

6.4 COMPONENTS OF ATM

Regardless of the cause of illness, there is a solution in ATM, which seeks to strike a balance between the patients' body, soul, and spirit. As shown in Figure 6.1, African traditional medicine is a holistic healthcare system that has three components or levels of specialty: divination, spiritualism, and herbalism [9].

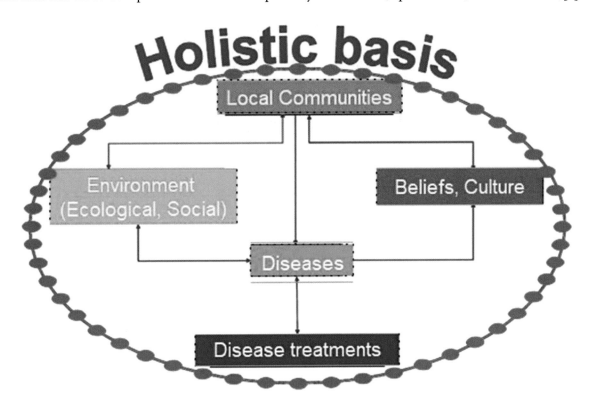

Figure 6.1 African traditional medicine is a holistic healthcare system.

- *Spiritualism:* ATM has spiritual and non-spiritual components. Africans have a unique way of understanding the visible world around them and the invisible, supernatural world of spirits, powers, and diseases. Illnesses and diseases are often regarded as having both natural and supernatural causes; they must be treated by physical and spiritual means including divination, incantations, animal sacrifice, exorcism, and herbs. Diseases are mostly attributed to witchcraft/sorcery, gods or immortal ancestors, or nature. Illness is believed to be related to supernatural causes such as angered spirits, witchcraft, or evil spirits. If the cause of the disease is perceived to be spiritual, the healer may use talisman, charm, amulets, and a spiritual bath to drive the evil spirits away from the victim. The spiritual healer may be diviners or fortune tellers, who may be seers, alfas, and priests.

- *Divination:* African spirituality sometimes involves diviners. Divination entails consulting the spirit world or communicating with the spiritual forces, such as the ancestors, spirits, and deities. It is regarded as a way to access information that is normally beyond the reach of the rational mind. Sacrifices are often offered at the request of the spirits, gods, and ancestors. During the colonial rule, traditional diviner-healers were outlawed and divination was declared illegal because they were regarded as practicing magic and witchcraft Some Christians also find divination as superstitious, incomprehensible, and unacceptable.

- *Herbal Medicine:* This is the non-spiritual component of ATM. For centuries, man has used plants as the primary therapeutic agent in medicine. The use of medicinal plants is a fundamental component of the African traditional medicine. Today, about 65% of the world's population relies on medicinal plants as an integral part of their healthcare. We will discuss more about African herbal medicine in the next section.

6.5 HERBAL MEDICINE

The use of traditional herbal medicine has a very long historical background that corresponds to the Stone Age. Herbal medicine is the cornerstone of African traditional medicine. It has been an integral part of the African healthcare system since time immemorial. According to the WHO, the goal of "health for all" cannot be achieved without the incorporation of herbal medicines in primary healthcare system.

In Africa, indigenous plants play an important role in treating various diseases. African traditional medicine across the continent extensively uses plant extracts which are believed to be efficacious. The leaves and fruits are the most commonly used plant parts to bring about cures. Herbalism is the application of herbs, roots, leaves, and other botanical products for treatment. Herbal medicine includes herbs, herbal preparations, and finished herbal products that contain parts of plants or other plant materials as active ingredients. Figure 6.2 shows some herbal medications [10]. Most of the herbs commonly used for the prevention and treatment of various illnesses are easily accessible, affordable, and available to the local community and well tolerated by the patients, with minimal side effects.

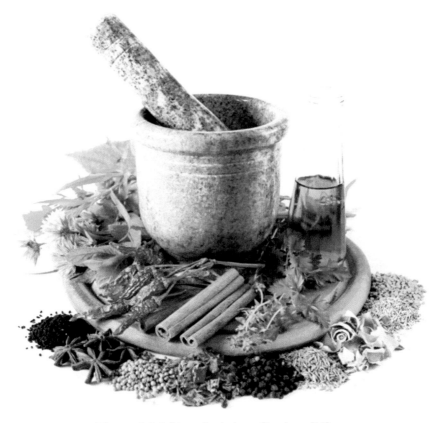

Figure 6.2 African herbal medications [10].

Traditional healers, also known as the herbalist in this case, often prescribe medicinal plants or herbs [11]. A typical African traditional healer is shown in 6.3 [8].

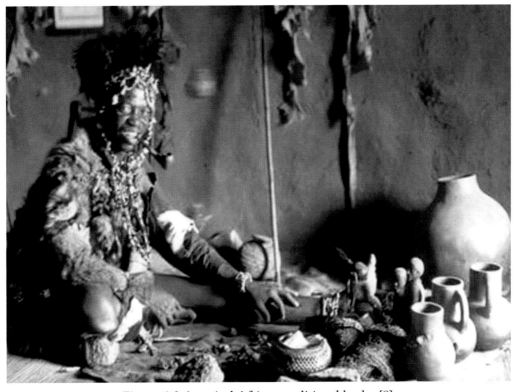

Figure 6.3 A typical African traditional healer [8].

Africa is endowed with many plants that can be used for medicinal purposes. Some of the plant parts and derivatives used in African traditional medicines are listed as follows [4,12]:

- *Roots:* The fleshy or woody roots of many African plant species are medicinal. Most of the active ingredients are usually sequestered in the root bark rather than the woody inner part.
- *Bulbs:* A bulb is an underground structure made up of numerous leaves of fleshy scales, e.g., Allium sativa (garlic) and Allium cepa (onions).
- *Rhizomes:* Woody or fleshy underground stem that grows horizontally and brings out their leaves above the ground, e.g., Zingiber officinale (ginger), which is used for respiratory problems; Imperata cylindrica (spear grass) for potency in men and Curcuma longa (turmeric), an antioxidant, anti-inflammatory, and anticancer drug.
- *Tubers:* Swollen fleshy underground structures which form stems/roots, e.g., potatoes and yams such as Dioscorea dumetorum for diabetes and Gloriosa superba for cancer.
- *Bark:* This is the outer protective layer of the tree stem or trunk. It contains highly concentrated phytochemicals with profound medicinal properties. A host of plants have barks of high medicinal value.
- *Gum arabic:* This is used extensively in organic products and is a food additive. It is also used widely as an ingredient in foods like candies and soft drinks.
- *Cannabis sativa:* The fresh leaves are made into a decoction that is taken three times a day to treat asthma. It is also used as steam.
- *Carduus tenuiflorus:* The plant is used to extricate poison or diseases from a sick person. It is believed the plant sucks out the cause of the illness in itself.
- *Datura stramonium:* Fresh leaves are used as a bandage that soothes pain and swelling. It is also used as an antiseptic after circumcision.
- *Emex australis:* This root is used on infants suffering from restlessness or constipation. It is used as a root decoction. Adults also use the decoction to treat constipation.
- *Lantana camara:* This is used to treat abdominal pains. The roots are boiled in water and drunk as tea twice a day. Also, it is used to treat urinary problems caused by sexual intercourse.
- *Opuntia ficus-indica:* This is used to treat sores between toes and the fingers.. The fresh leaf is baked in an open fire, the inner jelly is then used to apply on the sores.
- *Schinus molle:* The leaf decoction is taken orally to treat fever and influenza. The leaves are added to boiling water and the steam used to treat fever.
- *Anredera cordifolia:* The plants' leaves are crushed and applied on swollen feet whose cause is attributed to poor blood circulation. It is also used to treat kidney or liver problems.
- *Argemone mexicana:* This root decoction is administered through the use of an enema to cure kidney pain. The mixture should be used immediately, if left to stand for long it becomes harmful.
- *Bidens pilosa:* It is used to treat infertility in women. The roots are cleaned, boiled in water then taken orally.
- *Sutherlandia:* This provides immune system support against chronic diseases or immune deficiency diseases. It aids in reducing waste due to illnesses such as cancer, TB and aids. It regulates and stabilizes blood sugar levels.
- *Vernonia mespilifolia:* This is a shrub of the Asteraceae family used in the South African traditional medicine system for the management of weight loss, hypertension, and heartwater disease

- *Piper guineense:* This occurs commonly in West Africa where it is used for fungal infections instead of the costly and not always accessible conventional antifungals.
- *Shea butter:* This is the fat extracted from the nuts of shea trees (Vitellaria paradoxa). It has been used for its anti-inflammatory properties and for various dermatologic purposes including the treatment of boils, small wounds, cracks, crevices, and ulcers on the skin.

Preparing herbal medicines may vary around the continent. Common methods of preparation include extraction, mixing, infusions, and ashing. The sick person is often counseled by the herbalist on the dos and don'ts of treatment.

6.6 TRADITIONAL MEDICINE FROM SELECTED NATIONS

ATM has evolved over centuries of years. It has continued to receive increasing acceptance in African nations. Its practices vary significantly from country to country, and from region to region within Africa. The following nations are representative of the practice of ATM in some African nations.

- *South Africa:* In South Africa, there is currently a dual healthcare systems: one based on traditional medicine and another based on Western medical practice. The traditional healthcare system offers a cheap, individualized, and culturally appropriate alternative to the costly Western medicine. African traditional medical practitioners are extensively used in South Africa and are an indispensable component of the national healthcare system. South Africa consists of a wide diversity of tribes which is reflected in the way medicine is practiced. It has a rich tropical and temperate flora, harboring approximately 24,000 species. In South Africa, almost 60% of the population consults traditional healers, in preference to modern medical doctors. This is large reliance on the traditional medicine due to a number of factors: accessibility to the plants, affordability, conveniently located within the community, and extensive local knowledge among the local communities. The South African medicinal plant trade is a thriving at grassroots level. Medicinal plants are commonly sold at informal street markets or indoor shops. A large portion of South African medicinal plants have not been scientifically validated [13]. South Africa has significant progress in institutionalizing African traditional medicine and integrating traditional and complementary medicine.
- *Nigeria:* ATM practitioners provided the earliest medical care in Nigeria. The various ethnic groups in Nigeria have different healthcare practitioners beside their western counterparts. The Yorubas call them "babalawos," the Igbos call them "dibia," while the Northerners or Hausas call them "boka" [9]. Although healthcare in Nigeria is largely based on the modern medicine, the traditional health care is alive and well in both rural and urban areas because African traditional healers provide cheap, affordable, and accessible healthcare services [14]. Integrating or harmonizing traditional medicine with modern medicine has contributed immensely to the development of healthcare delivery in Nigeria.
- *Ghana:* Ghanaians believe in the physical and spiritual aspects of healing. Herbal spiritualists are known as "*bokomowo*" and are common all over the nation. They deal with in occult practices, divinations, incantations, and prayers. Taboos are part of African traditional religion. They are essentially things or behavior that are forbidden by a community. Although most Ghanaians

accept modern science-based medicine, traditional medicine is usually the first approach to treat any illness, especially in the rural areas. Lack of access to medical facilities, financial situation, education, not having enough medical doctors dictate type of healthcare they select [9].

- *Zambia*: The traditional medicine in Zambia is an interaction between biomedicine, Christianity, and an indigenous system. Christianity is part of traditional medicine developing in Zambia today. The term *ng'anga* is widely used to denote "doctors" in an indigenous sense. *Ng'anga* was perceived as an administrative nuisance for the colonial government, frowned upon as characteristically oriented towards belief in occult, witchcraft, and spirits. Regulation of *ng'anga* practice has not led to the prospect of their integration in to national healthcare [15].
- *East Africa*: ATM has been used by traditional health practitioners in East Africa (mainly in Kenya, Uganda and Tanzania) for management of diseases. There is widespread use of Aloe species in traditional healing practices in East Africa for various diseases. These species contain various carbohydrate polymers, particularly glucomannans. Traditional healers have adequate knowledge of Tod*dalia asiatica* and its uses. This medicinal plant is widely available and used in East Africa to manage malaria related symptoms. Malaria and malaria-related morbidity and mortality are important public health problems [16].

The traditional medicine practice in these African regions shows significanct differences between the nations in the degree of organization and integration of traditional medicine into mainstream health systems. Figure 6.4 shows some African nations that have national policies on traditional medicine [17].

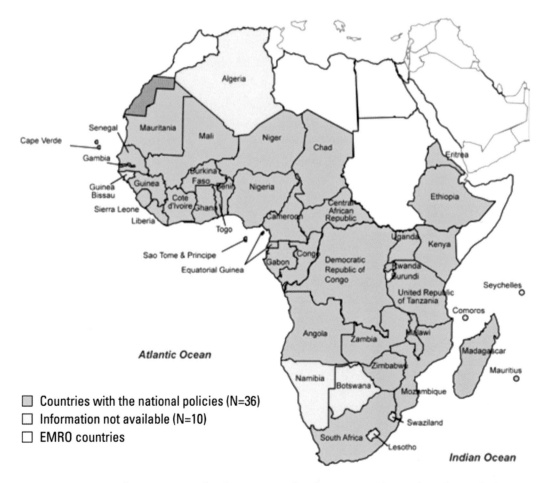

Figure 6.4 African nations that have national policies on traditional medicine [17].

6.7 REGULATION OF TRADIONAL MEDICINE

Health, safety, quality, and efficacy are universal concerns with regards to the regulatory requirements of traditional medicine. Inappropriate methods of collection, processing, and storage have all contributed to the negative impact of African medicine. Medicinal plant products may be contaminated with pollution, pesticides, microbial contaminants, heavy metals, and adulterants.

The absence of regulation of the medicinal plant trade in aspects such as collection, processing, and storage prevents African natural plant products from competing well in international markets. The regulation of traditional medicinal plant use embodies three fundamental aspects: quality, safety, and efficacy. The quality of medicinal plants varies considerably across nations. Good agricultural practice (GAP) is the first step in ensuring quality [18]. The safety of many herbal medicines has recently become a concern. ATM should be made as safe as possible because of the large numbers of people who use it. The traditional medicines claims to treat or cure HIV/AIDS effectively. There is need for research in order to improve the efficacy of ATMs.

6.8 APPLICATIONS OF ATM

For many generations, traditional medicine has been used to prevent and treat many diseases across Africa. In rural Africa, it is the only form of treatment that exists. Traditional healers are an important part of the traditional healthcare systems throughout Africa. The following are typical diseases that ATM has been able to treat.

- *Malaria:* Malaria is one of the most common diseases in the world, especially in the tropics. It remains one of the main causes of mortality among young children in sub-Saharan Africa. The symptoms of malaria include fever, headaches, etc. Traditional treatments to cure malaria have been investigated by numerous teams. Traditional healers for the treatment of malaria commonly use five plants originating from Ivory Coast: *Alchornea cordifolia, Mitragyna inermis, Nauclea diderrichii, Pterocarpus santalinoides,* and *Terminalia glaucescens* [19]. For each plant, three extracts were prepared in order to develop putative antiplasmodial compounds.
- *COVID-19:* After originating in China December 2019, COVID-19 has spread to at least 187 nations. Experts across Africa met and focused on the role of traditional medicine in the COVID-19 response. During the COVID-19 pandemic, ATM took the spotlight, starting with a widespread discussion of COVID-organics from Madagascar as a potential remedy for the virus. Tanzania produced its own famous herbal medicine to cure COVID. It is now famous for being one of the nations to declare itself COVID-free [20].
- *Diabetes:* Diabetes mellitus is a chronic disease affecting glucose metabolism. Two types of diabetes are differentiated: Type 1 and Type 2. Patients with Type 1 diabetes produce little or no insulin and are referred to as insulin-dependent. Patients with Type 2 diabetes do not respond normally to insulin due to insulin resistance and are referred to as non-insulin-dependent diabetes. Diagnosis of diabetes by traditional healers is mostly done by divination and herbal medicines. The most common herbal active ingredients used today in treating diabetes mellitus are flavonoids, tannins, phenolic, and alkaloids [21].

- *Women Disease/ Gynaecology*: A substantial number of African women seek treatment from traditional healers for a variety of problems, such as female reproductive, genital organs, infertility, abortion, to prevent abortion, contraception, breast and uterine cancer, and menstruation. Some traditional herbal remedies are used to treat gynaecological problems and disorders [22].
- *Depression:* This is a recurrent, life-threatening disorder with a diverse group of symptoms. It is a serious disorder with an estimate of lifetime prevalence as high as 20%. Out of 34 plants used for treatment of depression, only four plants are very effective antidepressant. The four plants, Agapanthus campanulatus, Boophone distica herb, Mondia whitei Skeels, and Xysmalobium undulatum, are used in southern Africa to treat mental illnesses related to depression [23].
- *Mental Illness:* The majority of the population in Africa use traditional healthcare to treat various mental conditions. The traditional healers use indigenous knowledge, beliefs, practices, and experiences in the diagnosis, treatment, and prevention of physical and mental illnesses. They provide culturally tailored treatment that holistically takes into account the importance of mind-body-spirit [24].

Other diseases that ATM has treated include HIV/ AIDS, convulsions, fever, headache, heartburn, pain, indigestion, boils, allergies, appetite stimulant, blood diseases, asthma, childbirth difficulties, cholera, cancers, epilepsy, psychiatric disorders, skin cancer, etc.

6.9 TRADITIONAL AND MODERN MEDICINE

Western or modern medicine is the conventional approach to medicine in western nations. Its therapy is based on allopathic principles. In Western medicine, the traditional view that illness was caused by spiritual forces is no longer popular. Although modern medicine has been successful in developed nations, it does not have the same positive impact in many developing African nations because hospitals and medical facilities are difficult for many Africans to get to due to poor road and transportation systems. Modern medicine can be too expensive and affordable for the average African [25].

Traditional African medicine often carries the perception and stigma of being irrational and ungrounded in scientific evaluation. Medicinal plant are incorrectly understood as reflecting superstition with no scientific basis [26]. Some critics argue that subjecting African traditional medicines to scientific research would be tantamount to a form of colonization and imperialism [27].

The WHO Traditional Medicines Strategy 2002–2005 provided a framework for action to promote the use of TM and Complementary Alternative medicine (TM/ CAM) in reducing mortality and morbidity in impoverished nations. The strategy had the following four objectives [28]:

- To integrate TM/CAM into national health care systems, where appropriate, by developing and implementing national TM/CAM policies and programs.
- To promote the safety, efficacy, and quality of TM/CAM by expanding the knowledge base of these remedies and by providing guidance on regulatory and quality assurance standards.
- To increase the availability and affordability of TM/CAM where appropriate, focusing on poorer populations.
- To promote therapeutically sound use of appropriate TM/CAM by providers and consumer.

In its strategy for 2014–2023, the WHO encourages the development and modernization of ATM as an integral part of emerging healthcare systems. WHO has recognized the need to integrate the traditional medicine on the orthodox medicine. As illustrated in Figure 6.5, integrating ATM into modern medicine is a challenge [29].

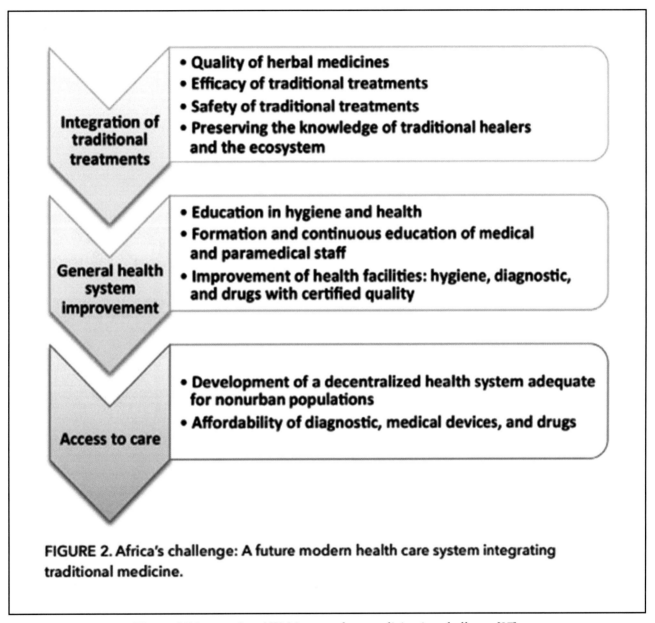

FIGURE 2. Africa's challenge: A future modern health care system integrating traditional medicine.

Figure 6.5 Integrating ATM into modern medicine is a challenge [27].

WHO has also developed model tools for institutionalizing African Traditional Medicine in health systems. National government can undertake the following actions in order to improve their traditional healthcare [30]:

• Develop policy, legal and regulatory frameworks for the practice of traditional medicine within the framework of national health policies and health legislation;

- Promote and conduct relevant scientific research on medicinal plants in collaboration with traditional health practitioners to validate claims made on safety, efficacy, and quality of traditional medicines.
- Ensure that intellectual property rights are priority items on the agenda of Member States to protect indigenous knowledge about traditional medicine.
- Establish an enabling economic, regulatory, and political environments for local production of traditional medicines as well as develop industries that can produce standardized remedies to increase access.
- Disseminate appropriate information to the general public to empower them with knowledge and skills for the proper use of traditional medicines.
- Build human and material resource capacity in order to carry out and accomplish institutionalization strategies.

6.10 BENEFITS

The use of medicinal plants has increased significantly in developed nations such as United States, Canada, Europe, and Australia with the predominant perception that herbal medicines are harmless and free of side effects [24]. African traditional medicine has been increasingly used by various communities in Africa and beyond due to its efficacy and increasing awareness. It is beneficial for therapy. Traditional healers in rural areas are beneficial because they are conveniently located within the community. ATM provides a platform through which cultural heritages are preserved. ATM will remain as a part of the healthcare option available to Africans. Other benefits include the following:

- *Affordability:* The majority of the African populations rely on ATM because it is readily accessible and is affordable. For most people living in rural areas, traditional medicines are the only available, easily accessible, and affordable source of healthcare.
- *Alternative Treatment:* Since modern medicine cannot cure all diseases, traditional medicine can intervene in the areas where modern medicine is weak or does not exist. It provides an alternative for the majority of Africans who cannot afford modern medical care. It provides solutions to some ailments (such as malaria, epilepsy, madness, and/or HIV/AIDS) that lack effective modern medical treatment. This have made the practice to be very lucrative. Many Africans prefer TM due to lack of trust on western medicine. Some are so skeptical to try western medicine.
- *Holistic Treatment:* ATM is a form of holistic healthcare system organized into three levels of specialty: divination, spiritualism, and herbalism. It seeks to strike a balance between the patients' body, soul and spirit. African herbal medicine is "holistic" in the sense that he sees the patient as consisting of the soul, spirit, and body.

6.11 CHALLENGES

Just like Western medicine, African traditional medicine faces some challenges. The dosage is often vague and the medicines are prepared under unhygienic conditions. Only a few of the African traditional medicinal plants have robust scientific and clinical proofs. There is still a scarcity of information addressing their active ingredients/constituents, quality assurance, efficacy, and standardization. ATM is not rooted in modern science, but is transmitted by the herbalists from one generation to another. In the process, some keys ingredients are lost or not documented. The literature and knowledge on African traditional medicine are highly scattered. Health insurance coverage is very difficult to justify if traditional medicine products and practices are not evidence based.

Other challenges include [9]:

- *Adverse Effects:* Herbal medicines may a have the potential to induce adverse effects if used incorrectly or in overdose. This may cause harm. The likelihood of adverse effects becomes more apparent due to indiscriminate, irresponsible, or nonregulated use and lack of proper standardization. These concerns have been the focus of many international forums on medicinal plants research and publications.

- *Toxic Effects:* As with most therapeutic drugs, there is a potential to cause toxicity. Several herbal medicines may have toxic effects. The toxic constituents from these plants can harm the human body systems such as cardiovascular system, digestive system, urinary system, immune system, muscular system, nervous system, reproductive system, etc. Unfortunately, most users of herbal medicines appear to be ignorant of their potential toxicity.

- *Inaccurate Diagnosis:* A major concern in using traditional herbal medicines is the possibility of being diagnosed inaccurately. An inaccurate diagnosis can be detrimental to a person's health.

- *Quality Control:* The major barriers to using of African medicinal plants are their poor quality control and safety. One major constraint to the growth of a African traditional medicine is the lack of technical specifications and quality control standards. Without effective quality control, consistency, and market value of the herbal product may be compromised. There is the challenge of ensuring the safety and efficacy of herbal medicines, and the quality of the source of raw materials. Investigations should address procedures for adopting for quality assurance and standardization of herbal products.

- *Lack of Regulation:* Due to lack of regulation, many people have begun to sell fraudulent products. Sometimes, it is so hard to distinguish genuine medicines from fakes. Some people sell fake traditional medicines on the streets with no one to be held accountable.

- *Lack of Scientific Validity:* The lack of scientific validity has definitely been an impediment. Aspects of African traditional medicine that cannot be proven by science (such as spiritism, psychic healing, soothsaying, and divination) are not part of the training of the medical herbalists

- *Secrecy:* Secrecy still surrounds the use of the African traditional medications. Prescriptions and practices of traditional medicine tend to be very secretive and localized. Before attaining knowledge in traditional African medicine, one is often required to be initiated into a secret society. The healers is often reluctant to hand down their knowledge to anyone but trusted relatives and initiates. The mode of transmission of traditional medicine by word-of-mouth has hindered its progress. This causes an erosion of valuable traditional knowledge or lack of detailed documentation of the traditional knowledge.

- *Interactions:* There is the possibility of interactions between African traditional medicines and prescribed medicines. Some herbal products that are safe when used on their own may pose a risk when taken in combination with Western drug. These interactions happen at a metabolic level.

An example of drug interactions are the effects of grapefruit juice and alcohol on many prescribed medicines. These combinations should be avoided.

- *Translation:* Since Africans speak many languages, there is a need to transform traditional medicine from one culture to another. A big challenge is on the translation of African traditional medicines. Traditional indigenous knowledge of medicinal plant in many groups is yet to be explored.

These challenges are depicted in Figure 6.6. They are causing ATM to being left behind on all fronts. The challenges must be fully addressed and overcome in order to fully achieve the objective of regulation, standardization, and integration of ATM in Africa.

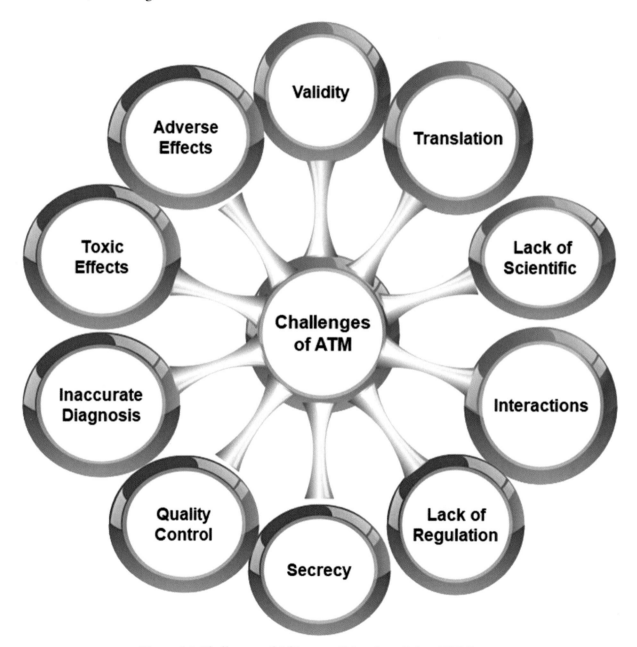

Figure 6.6 Challenges of African traditional medicine (ATM).

6.12 GLOBALIZATION OF ATM

The global trade in traditional medicines is increasing in both developing and developed nations. Although traditional medical practices are still in transition, it has a bright future which can be achieved through integration, harmonization, modernization, and standardization. The African traditional medicines, which was once described as primitive, is now globally recognized as mankind's saving grace. The pharmaceutical industry has come to realize the value of traditional medicine and now are collaborating with traditional healers on the medicinal effects of widely used plants.

As mentioned earlier, there are still many major challenges that need to be overcome and addressed for its full potential to be realized as the effective treatment of diseases. There is need for research in order to improve the efficacy of the African traditional medicine. African traditional medicine should improve and reach a stage where it can compete well with the Western medicines. To achieve this, some African nations are making concerted efforts to improve African traditional medicines through research. The World Health Organization (WHO) and the African Union (AU) are promoting scientific research into ATM.

The WHO has developed technical tools and guidelines to help African countries make traditional medicine an integral part of their health systems. It has been suggested that ATM should be considered the conventional medicine for Africa. In order for ATM to move to the next level, there is a need for improved collaboration between traditional practitioners and modern healthcare professionals. There is a need to integrate it on modern medicine. The future of African traditional medicine is bright considering increase of health care coverage, economic potential, and poverty reduction. Currently, there is a growing demand for TM in Europe, Asia and America.

6.13 CONCLUSION

African traditional medicine (ATM) refers to indigenous forms of healing that are practiced all over the continent of Africa. In 2001, during the African Union Summit, the Heads of State vowed that the forthcoming decade would incorporate the practice of African traditional medicine into their health care systems. Since 2003, 31 of August is celebrated as the African Traditional Medicine Day. This is to raise awareness of the critical role that traditional medicine plays in improving people's health.

Due the local demand of ATMs, it has been suggested that medical schools in Africa should include them in their curriculum as alternate medicines. Some universities such as Obafemi Awolowo University in Ile Ife, Nigeria, the University of Nigeria, Nsukka, Nigeria, and some institutions in Ghana and South Africa are already doing this [31,32]. Some efforts are being made to develop a unified indigenous knowledge systems database for ATM. More information on African traditional medicines can be found in numerous books in [1,33-54] and the following journals related to it:

- *Journal of Herbal Medicine*
- *Journal of Traditional Medicine & Clinical Naturopathy*
- *Journal of Ethnopharmacology.*
- *Journal of Traditional Medicine & Clinical Naturopathy*
- *African Journal of Traditional, Complementary and Alternative Medicines*
- *South African Medical Journal*

REFERENCES

[1]   V. Kuete (ed.), *Medicinal Plant Research in Africa.* Elsevier, 2013.

[2]   M. N. O. Sadiku, T. J. Ashaolu, and S. M. Musa, "African traditional medicine: A primer," *International Journal of Trend in Scientific Research and Development,* vol. 4, no. 4, 2020, pp. 123-127.

[3]   M. F. Mahomoodally, "Traditional medicines in Africa: An appraisal of ten potent African medicinal plants," *Evidence-Based Complementary and Alternative Medicine,* vol. 2013, 2013.

[4]   A. A. Abdullahi, "Trends and challenges of traditional medicine in Africa," *African Journal of Traditional, Complementary and Alternative Medicines,*vol, 8(S), 2011, pp. 115-123.

[5]   M. K. Asante, "Afrocentricity," April 2009,
http://www.asante.net/articles/1/afrocentricity/

[6]   R. C. Onwuanibe, "The philosophy of African medical practice," *A Journal of Opinion,* vol. 9, no. 3 (Autumn, 1979), pp. 25-28.

[7]   "Western medicine and African traditional health and social care essay," May 2016,
https://nursinganswers.net/essays/western-medicine-and-african-traditional-health-and-social-care-essay.php

[8]   P. Rasoanaivo, "African traditional medicines and indigenous knowledge systems,"
http://www.codata.info/10Conf/abstracts-presentations/Sessions%20H/H1/H1-Rasoanaivo.pdf

[9]   E. O. J. Ozioma and O. A. N. Chinwe, "Herbal medicine in African medicine," January 2019,
https://www.intechopen.com/books/herbal-medicine/herbal-medicines-in-african-traditional-medicine

[10]   "Herbal medicine – What are herbalists, herbal medications, and herbal treatments?" February 2019,'
https://the50shousewife.com/2019/02/05/herbal-medicine-what-are-herbalists-herbal-medications-and-herbal-treatments/

[11]   A. A. Adeyemi et al., "Traditional anti-fever phytotherapies in Sagamu and Remo North Districts in Ogun State, Nigeria," *Journal of Herbs, Spices & Medicinal Plants,* vol. 16, 2010, pp.3-4.

[12]   "Traditional African medicine," *Wikipedia,* the free encyclopedia,
https://en.wikipedia.org/wiki/Traditional_African_medicine

[13]   R. A. Street, W. A. Stirk, and J. V. Staden, "South African traditional medicinal plant trade—Challenges in regulating quality, safety and efficacy," *Journal of Ethnopharmacology,* vol. 119, no. 3, October 2008,pp. 705-710.

[14]   O. I. Isola, "The 'relevance' of the African traditional medicine (alternative medicine) to health care delivery system in Nigeria," *The Journal of Developing Areas,* vol. 47, no. 1, Spring 2013, pp. 319-338.

[15]   K. Sugishita, "Traditional medicine, biomedicine and Christianity in modern Zambia," *Journal of the International African Institute,* vol. 79, no. 3, 2009, pp.435-454.

[16]   J. A. Orwa et al., "The use of Toddalia asiatica (L) Lam. (Rutaceae) in traditional medicine practice in East Africa," Journal of Ethnopharmacology, vol. 115, 2008, pp. 257–262.

[17]   "Special issue: African traditional medicine,"
https://reliefweb.int/sites/reliefweb.int/files/resources/FCC3BB0257168C448525779000718FB3-who-ahm-special-issue-aug2010.pdf

[18] L. Gran, F. Sandberg, and K. Sletten,, "Oldenlandia affinis (R&S) DC: A plant containing uteroactive peptides used in African traditional medicine," *Journal of Ethnopharmacology*, vol. 70, no. 3, July 2000, pp. 197-203.

[19] "In South Africa, COVID-19 pits traditional medicine against clinical trial rules," December 2020, https://science.thewire.in/the-sciences/in-south-africa-covid-19-pits-traditional-medicine-against-clinical-trial-rules/

[20] Z. G. Ondo, "How traditional healers diagnose and treat diabetes mellitus in the Pretoria Mamelodi area and how do these purported medications comply with complementary and alternative medicine regulations," *Archives of Pharmacology and Therapeutics*, vol. 1, no. 2, 2019.

[21] V. Steenkamp, "Traditional herbal remedies used by South African women for gynaecological complaints," *Journal of Ethnopharmacology,* vol. 86, 2003, pp. 97–108.

[22] M. E. Pedersen et al., "Effects of South African traditional medicine in animal models for depression," *Journal of Ethnopharmacology*, vol. 119, 2008, pp. 542–548.

[23] L. Kajawu et al., "What do African traditional medical practitioners do in the treatment of mental disorders in Zimbabwe?" *International Journal of Culture and Mental Health,* vol. 9, no. 1, 2016, pp. 44-55,

[24] M. N. O. Sadiku, U. C. Chukwu, A. Ajayi-Majebi, and S. M. Musa, "Traditional medicine in Nigeria," International Journal of Trend in Scientific Research and Development, vol. 6, no. 3, April 2022, pp.1768-1775.

[25] J. F. Sobiecki, "The intersection of culture and science in South African traditional medicine," *Indo-Pacific Journal of Phenomenology,* vol. 14, no. 1, 2014, pp. 1-10,

[26] A. Nyika, "The ethics of improving African traditional medical practice: Scientific or African traditional research methods?" *Acta Tropica,* vol. 112, Supplement 1, November 2009, pp. S32-S36.

[27] M. E. Mothibe and M. Sibanda, "African traditional medicine: South African perspective," February 2019, https://www.intechopen.com/chapters/65475

[28] J. Kahumba et al., "Traditional African medicine: From ancestral knowledge to a modern integrated future," *Science,* vol. 350, 2015.

[29] A. A. Elujoba, O. M. Odeleye, and C. M. Ogunyemi, "Traditional medicine development for medical and dental primary health care delivery system in Africa," *African Journal of Traditional, Complementary and Alternative Medicines,* vol. 2, no. 1, 2005, pp.46-61

[30] A. Popat et al., "The toxicity of Callilepis laureola, a South African traditional herbal medicine," *Clinical Biochemistry,* vol. 34, no. 3, May 2001, pp. 229-236.

[31] M. Moeta et al., "Integrating African traditional health knowledge and practices into health sciences curricula in higher education: An Imbizo approach," *International Journal of African Renaissance Studies - Multi-, Inter- and Transdisciplinarity,* vol. 14, no.1, 2019, pp. 67-82.

[32] A. A. Okunade, "Traditional medicine and health care in transition," in N. S. Lawal, M. N. O. Sadiku, and P. A. Dopamu (eds.), *Understanding Yoruba Life & Culture.* Trenton, NJ: Africa World Press, 2004.

[33] M. A. Makinde, *African Philosophy, Culture, and Traditional Medicine.* Ohio University Press, 1988.

[34] H. D. Neuwinger, *African Traditional Medicine: A Dictionary of Plant Use and Applications. With Supplement: Search System for Diseases.* Stuttgart, Germany: Medpharm, 2000.

[35] P. I. Osuji, *African Traditional Medicine: Autonomy and Informed Consent.* Springer, 2014.

[36] M. Last and G. L. Chavunduka, *The Professionalisation of African Medicine*. Routledge, 2020.

[37] D. Daniel et al., *Traditional Medicine and Herbs of Africa*. Independently Published, 2020.

[38] M. Mackintosh et al., *Making Medicines in Africa: The Political Economy of Industrializing for Local Health*. Palgrave Macmillan, 2016.

[39] N. Gqaleniand and N. Mbatha, *African Traditional Medicine At the Cross Roads in South Africa Challenges Faced by Its Institutionalization*. Smashwords, 2018.

[40] I. W. Zartman, *Traditional Cures for Modern Conflicts: African Conflict Medicine."* Boulder, CO: Lynne Rienner Publishers, 2000.

[41] Z. Yaniv and U. Bachrach (eds.), *Handbook of Medical Plants*. Binghamton, NY: Haworth Press, 2005.

[42] M. M. Iwu, *Handbook of African Medicinal Plants*. Boca Raton, FL: CRC Press, 2nd edition, 2014.

[43] N. Mbatha et al., *African Traditional Medicine at the Cross-Roads in South Africa: Challenges Faced by its Institutionalization*. Nompumelelo Mbatha and Nceba Gqaleni, 2018.

[44] U. F. Adamu, *Modern and Traditional Medicine: Conflicts and Reconciliation*. Nigeria: Safari, 2013.

[45] C. Wambebe, *African Indigenous Medical Knowledge and Human Health*. Boca Raton, FL: CRC Press, 2018.

[46] C. N. Chacha and I. Sindiga (eds.), *Traditional Medicine in Africa (Sparrow Reader Series)*. East African Educ. Publ., 1997.

[47] T. Gyatso and C. Hakim, *Essentials of Tibetan Traditional Medicine*. North Atlantic Books, 2010.

[48] H. Lowe, A. Payne-Jackson, and Cynthia Johnson, *The Legacy of African, American & Caribbean Traditional Medicines - Mind, Body, and Spirit*. Pelican Publishers Limited, 2009.

[49] H. C. Covey, *African American Slave Medicine: Herbal and non-Herbal Treatments*. Lexington Books, 2008.

[50] D.O. Oyebola, *African Traditional Medicine: Practices Among the Yoruba of Nigeria*. Christian Faith Publishing, 2019.

[51] I. W. Zartman (ed.), *Traditional Cures for Modern Conflicts; African Conflict "Medicine."* Lynne Rienner Publishers. 2000.

[52] P. O. Amanze, *African Traditional Medicine*. United Kingdom, AuthorHouse, 2011.

[53] L. Afrika, *The Textbook of African Holistic Health*. Llaila Afrika, 2018

[54] S. Mazaza, *Urban African Traditional Healers*. LAP Lambert Academic Publishing, 2009.

7

CHAPTER

Yoruba Traditional Medicine

"Work is the medicine for poverty." – Yoruba Proverb

7.1 INTRODUCTION

Health is regarded as order, while disease is disorder. The desire to have and sustain good health cuts across national, geographic, and political boundaries. Every culture has a means of escaping the possibility of illness. Medicine is meant to manage our health, treat illness, and cure diseases. Globally, each culture developed unique indigenous healing traditions based on by the culture, beliefs, and environment. Traditional medicine used to be the dominant medicine readily available to millions of people in Africa in both rural and urban communities. It is still generally available, affordable, and commonly used in large parts of Africa, Asia, and Latin America. According to the World Health Organization (WHO), traditional medicine is the sum total of all knowledge and practices used in diagnosis, prevention, and elimination of physical and mental diseases, relying on practical experience and observations handed down from generation to generation. It consists of all kinds of folk medicine that was handed down by the tradition of a community or ethnic group [1].

Traditional medicines include ethnomedical beliefs and traditions specific to individual cultures. They take various forms of therapies such as herbal medicine, vegetables, animals, mineral substances, homeopathy, mud bath, music therapy, wax bath, reflexology, dance therapy, hydrotherapy, mind and spirit therapies, self-exercise therapies, radiation and vibration, osteopathy, chiropractice, radiant heat therapy, therapeutic fasting, and psychotherapy [2]. The custodians of the various forms of traditional medicine are often referred to as traditional healers.

Yoruba is one of the three main ethnic groups, and the second most populous, in Nigeria. The Yoruba people of southwestern Nigeria have an impressive system of indigenous medicine. For the Yoruba, reality is rooted in both the physical and the spiritual realms. Although Christianity and Islam have somewhat replaced Yoruba traditional religions, the thoughts of the people about life are still shaped by the old worldview. Before the advent of modern medical practices, the Yoruba people sought healthcare from traditional healers, who were experts in the science of using barks, leaves, grasses, and roots to cure ailments and illnesses. The cost of modern medicine is rapidly increasing with improvements in technologies and in many cases is not affordable to people in developing nations. On the other hand, traditional medicines are widely available and affordable [3].

Yoruba traditional medicine (YTM) is a body of knowledge that has been developed and accumulated by Yoruba thousands of years ago. The Yorubas have relied on traditional herbal medicine to meet their healthcare needs. Numbering over 36 million people, the Yoruba live in the present-day republics of Nigeria, Benin and Togo. The Yorùbá people are one of the most researched ethno-linguistic groups in Africa. Their traditional medicine is essentially an African medical system practiced primarily in West Africa and the Caribbean. Although many Yoruba people have become Christians and Muslims, those who practice the traditional religion of their ancestors have managed to coexist peacefully with others.

This chapter introduces readers to Yoruba traditional medicine. It begins by providing a brief historical background for YTM. It discusses the concept of YTM. It considers some Yoruba herbs. It presents some typical applications of YTM. It highlights the benefits and challenges of the traditional Yoruba medicine. It covers the globalization of YTM. The last section concludes with comments.

1.2 BRIEF HISTORY OF YORUBA MEDICINE

The Yorùbá people, who inhabit a significant part of West Africa including Nigeria, have been practicing their unique set of religious customs for centuries. Their medical traditional practices developed within a culture that venerates ancestors. Their philosophy on health and healing cannot be divorced from their tradition and belief system. The orisas, or gods of the Yoruba, were former ancestors such as Oduduwa, the legendary ancestor of all Yoruba people. The orishas serve as the intermediaries between man and the supreme creator, known as Olodumare or Olorun. The Yoruba people often believe that sickness is a punishment of a god or ancestor, who must be placated by offering sacrifice. According to oral history, the Ifa Corpus was revealed by the mystic prophet, Orunmilla, around 4,000 years ago in the ancient city of Ile-Ife, the major city in Yorùbáland. Ọ̀rúnmìlà taught the people the customs of divination, prayer, dance, symbolic gestures,, and communal elevation. He was the first man to practice herbal medicine in Yorubaland. He was endowed with this knowledge by God. He also led the priesthood of Ifà. The Ifá Corpus is considered to be the foundation of the traditional medicine. The Yorùbá people do not begin any undertaking without first consulting Ifá. They believe that sickness can be caused by enemies (òtá), which include witchcraft (àjẹ), sorcery (osó), a god (òrìṣà), or ancestors (ẹbọra). There are also natural illnesses (ààrẹ) and hereditary diseases (àìsàn ìdílé).

Traditional healing among the Yoruba people remained popular during the colonial period between 1922 and 1955. The British colonial masters brought in conventional medicine to Nigeria. Now both systems of medicine exist side by side in the country; and they have the primary objective to cure, manage or prevent diseases and maintain good health. The interaction of the Yorùbá healing with Western medicine began in the middle of the nineteen century when missionaries first made contact with the Yorùbá people. However, during colonial rule, traditional beliefs and practices were discriminated against. The Yorùbá healing system was derogatorily deemed primitive and unscientific because of its ritualistic aspects.. The activities of missionaries and colonial governmental policies entailed attempts to do away with the Yorùbá healing system. Although many Yoruba people have become Christian and Muslim since colonization, those who practice the traditional religious beliefs of their ancestors have managed to coexist peacefully with their non-traditional neighbors. The YTM has survived into the modern age. The reason for the survival of Yorùbá healing system in spite colonialism and modernity rests largely on their resilient culture [4].

In post independence Nigeria, concerted efforts have been made to recognize traditional medicine as important component of healthcare delivery system. However, Western-trained physicians seem to unwilling to allow TM and their practitioners to be part in the official system of medical care. The concepts of change and continuity are relevant to understanding the evolution of TM in spite of "threats" of modernity in Nigeria.

7.3 CONCEPT OF YORUBA MEDICINE

Each culture has its set of ethnomedical beliefs and practices associated with health and illness. When adopted outside its traditional culture, traditional medicine is often classified as a form of alternative medicine (AM). Traditional medicines are sources of relatively inexpensive drugs for diagnosis and treatment of illness and diseases. Just like the orthodox medicines, traditional medicines have the primary objective to cure, manage or prevent diseases and maintain good health. Yoruba traditional African medicines are beneficial in treating disease or maintaining good health.

The Yoruba people developed a form of holistic healthcare system organized into three levels of divination, herbalism, and spiritualism. Divination is basically consulting the spirit world. Herbalism (also Herbal medicine) is the study and the use of medicinal plants, which is the cornerstone of Yoruba traditional medicine. Traditional medicine has always been linked to spiritualism or spirituality. The Yorubas regard illness and disease as something connected to spirits, witches, wizards or ancestors. Thus, the YTM practices utilize both herbalism (practiced herbal healers) and divination (practiced by the priests of Ifa) [5]. It is commonly believed that YTM started from a religious text, called *Ifa Corpus*. Ifá divination is often used to diagnose and treat illnesses. As shown in Figure 7.1, Ifá divination is a common means of diagnosing and treating chronic illnesses among the Yoruba people [6]. The Ifa priest is often called Babalawo, the diviner-priest. One can only become a Babaláwo after years of rigorous training. Exorcism can also be performed by a religious leader or a priest. This is a practice of expelling demons or evil spirits from people who are possessed.

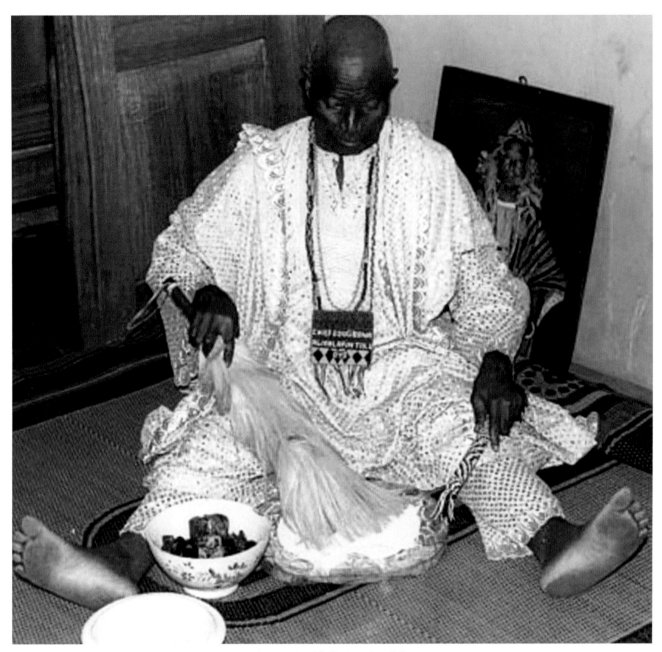

Figure 7.1 Ifa divination [6].

The Yoruba traditional medicines, known as *oogun* or *oogun ibile,* are usually made from natural substances and include botanical matter, crystals, metal, particular animal skins, claws, and teeth. Yoruba land is home to an extensive and diverse medicinal plant life. Figure 7.2 shows some typical herbs, roots, and plants can have health benefits [7]. Traditional medicines can be used in various ways. Sometimes the preparations of medicine is done by burning the ingredients into powder and then rubbing the powder over the affected part of the body. Some preparations are made by cooking the ingredients as soup. Sometimes pepper soup is used mostly to cure a cold, catarrh, allergies, and a loss of appetite. Traditional chemical products are also used in southwestern Nigeria as traditional adornment especially for wedding and funerals. The medicines are easily available at a street-side pharmacy, almost anywhere in Nigeria.

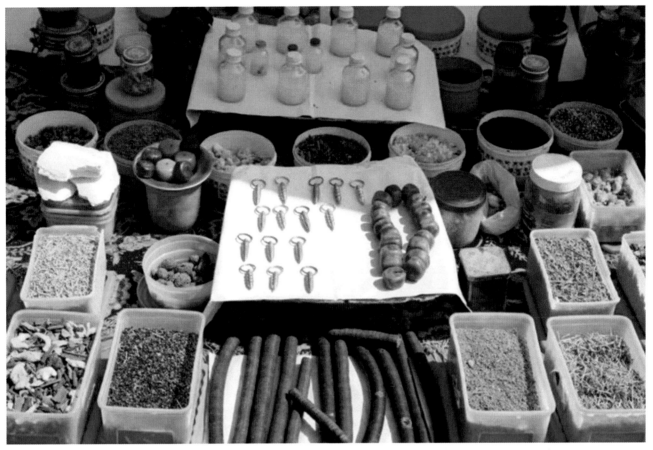

Figure 7.2 Typical herbs, roots, and plants on display for health benefits [7].

The traditional medical practitioner is always interested in the spiritual causes of illness. He believes that a person has two parts: body and soul. Understanding the spiritual causes of the disease will help him placate the negative forces and then propose appropriate treatment for the patient. The medicines are related to Yoruba religion in terms of rituals, taboos, divination, and the supernatural. Traditional healers usually receive formal training before they start to practice.

One may be tempted to call the more spectacular aspects of Yoruba traditional medicine as magic, but it is not. Magic is when you do not understand the technology. The forces behind the technology may be elusive or hard to understand, they are still identifiable. The spiritual technology of traditional Ifa medicines requires rules to follow. The rule may be the correct chanting of a correct incantation. If the proper rules for the medicines are not followed, one will have disappointing results because the medicine will most likely not work. Medicines or magic was classified into protective and harming medicines [8]. There were also medicines for fevers, colds, pregnancy, etc.

7.4 YORUBA HERBS

Medicinal herbs play tremendous roles in human history and medical treatment. Herbal medicine (also known as botanical medicine) is an important component of Yoruba of traditional medicine. The Yorubaland is home to an extensive and diverse medicinal plant life. The term *agbo* is the Yoruba name for herbs in a variety of forms and concoctions. It usually comes as liquid, pastries, syrups or crushed mixtures of different things such as the bark, leaves, stems, and roots of trees. Herbs can be added into foods, teas, and beauty products. The use of medicinal plants (either alone or in combination with other herbs) for treating diseases has become popular in recent years and they continue to play a crucial role in human health. Herbs can help to ensure wellness, boost immunity, encourage restful sleep, enhance alertness, reduce stress, and increase antioxidant intake [9]. People use herbs because they are cheaper and works faster than the conventional medicines. Some medical experts caution and discourage people from using the herbs because they believe that their preparations are dangerous to human health [10]. Since herbalism is a complex science that stems from traditions, cultures, and worldviews, consulting a qualified herbalist is the safest, most effective way to use herbs.

Some herbs in Yoruba culture include the following [12-14]:

- "Osun" (cam wood): When applied to the skin, the rough texture of the ground cam wood possibly causes epidermabrasion which results in the removal of dead skin tissue, encouraging new cell production.
- "Ori" (shea butter): This made from the fruit of the shea butter tree. The stem of the shea butter tree is also used to make a mortar. The oils extracted from the tree act as an emollient and help to keep the skin soft.
- "Tiro" (local eyeliner): This is antimony, which comes as shiny silver-like pieces. When ground with a piece of charcoal, it can be applied to the eyelashes.
- "Obi" (kola nut): This is the fruit of the kola tree. It plays a significant role in Yoruba culture. No wedding can be completed without kola nuts.
- "Ewuro" (bitter leaf): This bitter leaf is a remedy for stomach ache. It is also used for treating malaria, typhoid fever, and diarrhea. It has strong medicinal properties that help to clear the blood and lymphatic system of impurities. Healing is done using herbs like bitter leaves, shown in Figure 7.3 [11].

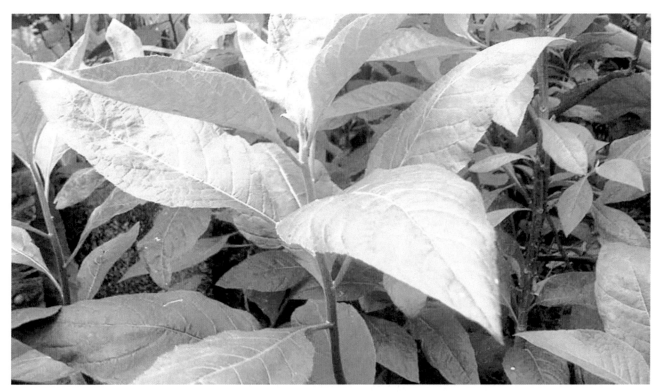

Figure 7.3 Bitter leaves anti-diabetic medication [11].

- "Orogbo" (bitter kola nuts): These are used as a remedy for throat infections, chest colds, bronchitis, sexual performance, and liver disorders. Figure 7.4 displays some bitter kola nuts [11]. This is an easy way to increase your sperm. This element of Yoruba wedding symbolizes the health of the future family.

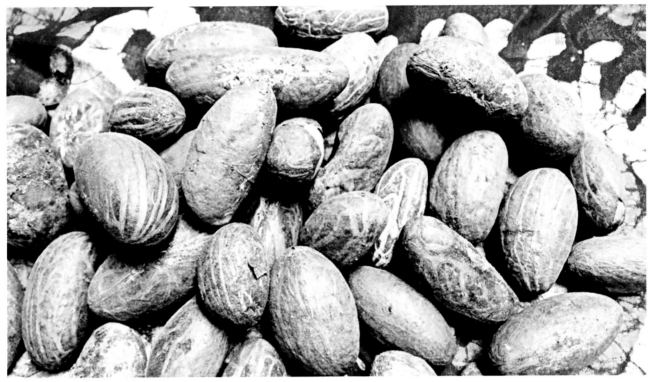

Figure 7.4 Bitter kola nuts used as a remedy for throat infections, chest colds, bronchitis, and sexual performance [11].

- "Ewe ile" (moringa oleifera): This is a popular flowering tree. It is referred to as the miracle tree. Moringa is used for too many purposes such as culinary, cosmetic, and medicinal uses. It is rich in amino acids, minerals, and vitamins especially vitamin A, C, and E.
- Aloe vera: This leaf is commonly used to treat constipation and skin diseases. Its gel is used as a home remedy for accelerating the healing of burn injuries. It is also used sometimes as traditional medicine in diabetes management.
- "Efirin" (scent leaf): This is a popular medicinal plant in the Yorubaland. It is commonly used as a home remedy for diarrhea, dysentery, stomach ache, and vomiting. It is also used for preventing and treating cold and catarrh, cough, fever, and malaria.
- "Efo Yarin" (wild lettuce): This is a widely used medicinal plant used in traditional medicine worldwide. The plant can be used to make a home remedy for pain relief, e.g., arthritic pain, colic pain, joint pain, muscle pain, and muscle spasms. It is also used for the treatment of insomnia because of its sedative properties.
- "Gbure" (water leaf): This is a very popular medicinal plant in Yorubaland and beyond. It medicinal uses include boosting the immune system of sick people, diarrhea, hepatitis, and liver enlargement. Waterleaf is also good for pregnant women and for making vegetable food.
- "Oyin" (honey): This is used in combination with different herbs. An example of a herbal remedy would be a mix of bitter leaf and basil to reduce high blood pressure.
- Alligator pepper is a traditional ingredient in many dishes in Yoruba cuisine and herbal preparation.

The list is by no means exhaustive. In the Yoruba culture, there is a thin line between cosmetic products and medicinal products. The herbs are used for medicinal purposes, as food spices, bodily adornment, and also for fragrances or perfumes. There are many forms in which herbs can be administered; the most common form is a liquid consumed as herbal tea. As shown in Figure 7.5, the herbal sellers play a functional role in providing healthcare at the primary health care level in Nigeria [15].

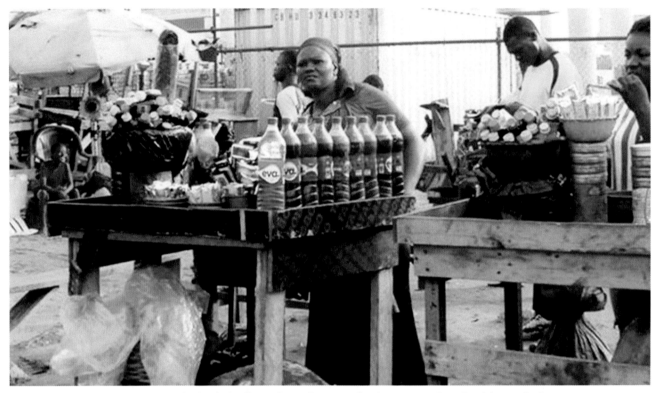

Figure 7.5 The herbal sellers play a functional role in providing healthcare [16].

7.5 APPLICATIONS OF YORUBA MEDICINE

From ancient times, the continent of Africa has always provided solutions to multi-faceted sickness and problems of human race. The Yoruba traditional medicines are undeniably beneficial in preventing and treating disease or maintaining good health. Many traditional healers (or native doctors) can use divination to find the causes of illness and know whether its origin was from a physical or spiritual treatment. By experience, diagnosis is reached through spiritual means and a treatment is prescribed, usually consisting of a herbal remedy. Traditional healers employ a variety of treatments including fasting, dieting, herbal therapies, bathing, massage, and surgical procedures. Some traditional healers use charms, incantations, and the casting of spells in their treatments [16]. They are strongly convinced that they can cure or treat almost every ailment including headaches, fevers, pains, arthritis, wounds, skin infections, women infertility, cancer, stroke, erectile dysfunction, gonorrhoea. insomnia, convulsion, urinary tract infection, diarrhea, high blood pressure, ringworm, diabetes, etc. The following illnesses are samples of what Yoruba traditional medicine can cure.

- *Malaria*: Malaria is a major disease in tropical regions of the world, It is a mosquito-borne disease that has a disproportionate effect in developing nations such as Nigeria. The search for malaria cure is the first focal area in the new drive for the use of traditional medicine in Nigeria, because of the high health risk due to malaria. Malaria has long been treated with plant-based medicine. Quinine, which comes from the bark of a cinchona tree, was first isolated as an antimalarial compound in the 1800s [17]. Over 1200 plant species from 160 families can be used to treat malaria and fever. A combination of garlic cloves, ginger roots, lemon grass, lime, onions, unripe pawpaw, and utazi boiled together is often consumed as both preventive and curative measures for malaria.

- *Fever:* Typhoid fever is currently a major health problem in developing nations with limited success of treatment with antimicrobial agent. Several studies have identified medicinal plants that are promising to act as potential agent that be effectively used to treat typhoid fever [18].

- *Erectile Dysfunction:* Inability to perform sexually is generally known as sexual dysfunction. It takes different forms including premature ejaculation, erectile dysfunction (ED), arousal difficulties, compulsive sexual behavior, orgasmic disorder, and failure of detumescence. ED is a sign of physical condition due to stress, relationship strain, low self-esteem, anxiety, depression, diabetes and reduced sexual interest. A major symptom of ED is a man's inability to keep an erection strong enough for sexual intercourse. Extracts from Tributus terrestris can be used for treatment [19]. Scientifically proven local herbal aphrodisiacs can be used for treating sexual dysfunction. An aphrodisiac is an agent (food or drug) that arouses sexual desire. Nigerian scientists have confirmed that eating moderate quantities of bitter cola (*orogbo*) is a good sexual performance medicine for men with ED. They have also patented eye drops made with bitter kola for preventing blindness in patients. Bitter kola is an easy way to increase sperm without going through any medical means.

- *Stroke:* An ancient herbal extract known as ginkgo biloba (herbal supplement) might benefit people who have experienced ischemic stroke. Most strokes are ischemic, wherein the artery that supplies blood to the brain becomes blocked, most commonly due to a blood clot.

- *High Blood Pressure*: High blood pressure (or hypertension) is the most common, preventable risk factor for heart disease. It is a serious condition that requires treatment to prevent more problems. It affects a lot of adults. It can be treated with medication, dietary, and lifestyle changes. High blood pressure is defined as having at least one of the following [20]:

> systolic blood pressure (the top number) over 130 mm Hg
> diastolic blood pressure (the bottom number) over 80 mm Hg
> both systolic and diastolic values above these levels

Studies have shown that some herbs (such as Basil, Parsley) and spices (such as garlic, cinnamon, ginger, and celery seeds) can be used to reduce blood pressure levels. Basil extracts can help relax blood vessels and thin the blood, which in turn helped reduce blood pressure in humans. Ginger is easy to incorporate into your diet with meals and it can likewise lower blood pressure and improve circulation. Cinnamon is effective in reducing blood pressure in humans by relaxing blood vessels. Garlic is rich for blood circulation and heart health.

- *Diarrhea:* This is regarded as a worldwide killer disease. It is essentially is a digestive condition in which faeces are passed from the bowels more frequently and in a liquid form. The leading cause of death from diarrhea is as a result of dehydration, whereby the body loses more water than it takes in. Factors contributing to diarrhea include poor sanitation, consumption of infected food or water, unclean environment, bacteria, viruses, excessive bowel movements, infected fomites, etc. Herbs such as peppermint tea, rosemary, chamomile, lemon, orange, fennel tea and catnip can help in curing diarrhea. *Cinnamomum tamala* is also commonly used for treating diarrhea [21].

- *Diabetes:* There is a continuous increase in the prevalence of diabetes cases. Major cause is our eating habits and sedentary lifestyle. Change of lifestyle and proper medical intervention can prevent progression to diabetes. Many herbs have been used to treat diabetes. For example, Yoruba herbs can be used to cure diabetes and its complications. Taken in moderation, the herbs can lower sugar level. Incorporating these herbs in our daily routine can surely help pre-diabetics stay healthy for longer time without progressing to type-2 [22,23].

- *Woman Infertility:* The Yoruba traditional healers are knowledgeable in the various diseases and medicines associated with women, pregnancy, and childbirth. The fear of infertility influences decision-making when it comes to using contraceptives, induced abortion, and pregnancy before marriage. The Yoruba women believe that infertility can be due to spiritual reason, for which modern medicine is not appropriate. They often seek treatment for infertility from local herbalists and spiritual specialists [24].

7.6 BENEFITS

The Yoruba have an impressive system of indigenous medicine. There is a lot of benefits for using Yoruba herbal medicine. The Ooni of Ife, the highest traditional king in Yorubaland shown in Figure 7.6, claimed that he does not use anything other than traditional products and has never been to the hospital to treat any sickness in recent times. He is a living testimony of the efficacy of local herbal products [25]. Yoruba herbal medicine is holistic in that it addresses issues of the soul, spirit, and body. Nigeria suffers from shortage of Western-trained healthcare practitioners and traditional medicine is the only means of healthcare available to a large portion of her population who live in the rural areas. If funds are released for research and development of traditional medicine practices and products, a nation will cut down the health budget drastically.

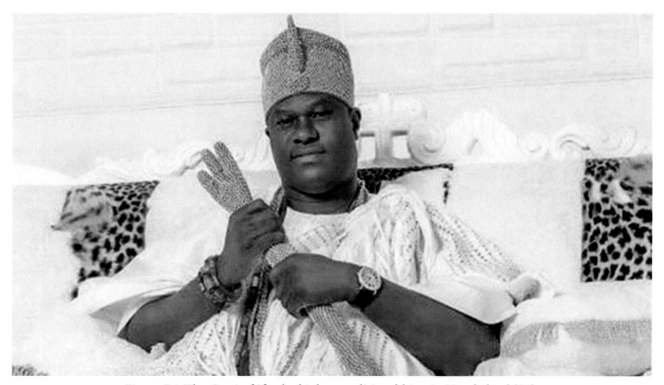

Figure 7.6 The Ooni of Ife, the highest traditional king in Yorubaland [24].

Other benefits of tradition medicine include [25]:

- *Cost Effective*: The high rate of poverty in Africa generally has made it difficult if not impossible for most Africans yo obtain Western medication when they are sick. Western healthcare is indeed expensive, and its delivery is slow. Traditional medicine is more affordable than conventional medicine. Yorùbá philosophy forbids profiteering from traditional healthcare delivery and this makes TM affordable to everyone.

- *No Prescription:* It is easier to obtain TM than prescription medicine. One does not need to see a doctor to get prescriptions before purchasing TM. It is easier to obtain herbal products and avoid additional healthcare costs.

- *Efficacy:* Herbs are used around the world for the treatment of various ailments such as cardiovascular disease, prostate problems, depression, inflammation, and weakened immune system. Many studies prove their efficacy.

- *Safety:* Herbal medicines are considered safe, effective, and beneficial by most users. The fact that herbs are of natural origin does not automatically guaranty their safety.

- *Diverse Health Practices:* Using traditional medicine provides significant advantages for treating many diseases. Yoruba traditional medicines are diverse health practices beliefs that incorporate plant, animal, spiritual therapies, manual techniques, and exercises which are applied to treat, diagnose or prevent illness. The leaves, stem, roots, and seeds of Yoruba plants have various culinary and medicinal benefits. Some plants have proven antibacterial and antifungal properties which makes them suitable for treating infections. TM is used for treating various diseases such as hypertension, stroke, insomnia, and convulsion.

- *Holistic Health*: Yorubic medicine is widely known as a traditional medical practice that is holistic in treatment. It tales into account one's body, mind, emotions, and spiritual life. It is organized into three levels of specialty: divination, spiritualism, and herbalism. Various techniques used include natural diet, herbal remedies, nutritional supplements, exercise, relaxation, psycho-spiritual counseling, meditation, breathing exercises, and other self-regulatory practices.

- *Unique Care:* There are some sickness (such as Yoruba mágùn) which cannot be detected nor diagnosed scientifically or Western-style machines because they are spiritual in nature. Such ailments require the attention of diviners who pry into the realm of the metaphysical. Herbal traditions empower individuals to study and work with herbs for their own health.

Some of these benefits are illustrated in Figure 7.7.

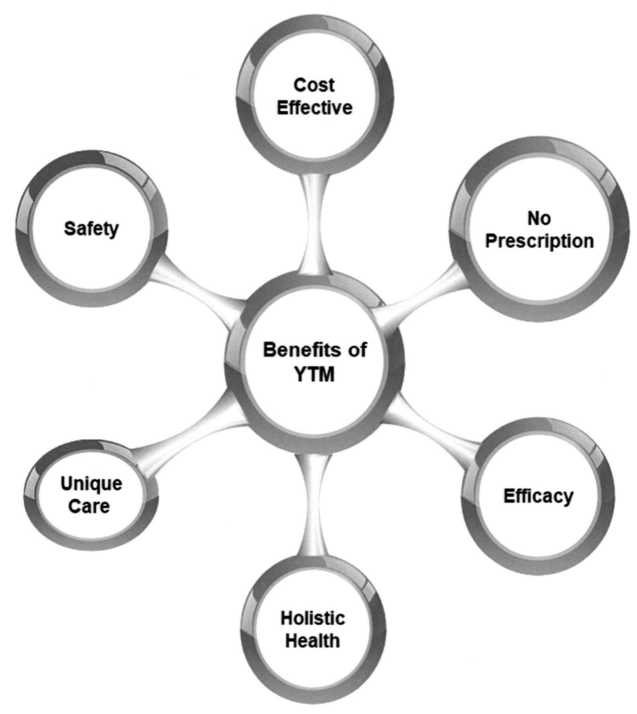

Figure 7.7 Benefits of Yoruba traditional medicine (YTM).

7.7 CHALLENGES

TM has a number of challenges which must be addressed in order for it to thrive. The composition for an herbal mixture is unknown and are not regulated, which is the major challenge. Other challenges include the following:

- *Safety of Herbal Medicines (HM):* The fact that herbs are of natural origin does not automatically guaranty their safety. It is necessary to evaluate the safety, efficacy, and quality of these preparations and products. The indiscriminate, unregulated use of herbal medicines (HM)may put the health of their users at risk of toxicity or overdose [26]. The medicines are prepared under unhygienic environment. The possible <u>adverse effects</u> of traditional medicines are not well documented

- *Secrecy:* Prescriptions of Yoruba traditional medicines are often secretive. They are based on knowledge passed from generation to generation of traditional healers. This can result in vague doses and can lead to severe health consequences. Indigenous knowledge is being lost every day due to lack of documentation caused by secrecy.

- *Interference:* This traditional remedy may interfere with the normal metabolism of drugs and the patients should understand the risks of interaction.

- *Toxicity:* This may arise due to herb-drug interaction. Incorrect identification and misuse of plants may also lead to toxicity. An important source of toxicity of herbal medicines is microbial contamination due to poor sanitary conditions during preparation.

- *Overdose:* It is difficult for people who take Yoruba medicine "agbo" (popular concoction prepared from a variety of herbs) to know the proper dose. Overdose or indiscriminate use of traditional concoctions can affect the multisystem functions of the kidney and liver.

- *Tensions with Western Medicine(WM):* Traditional medicine has a number of inherent challenges rooted in tensions with Western medicine (WM). It seems characterized by mysticism and magic. It remains a mystery and a mirage to much of the western world. Relegation of non-Western medicines to the unregulated nutraceutical industry is unsafe. The herbalists have no systematic way of classifying their drugs as in western medicine.

- *Integration:* There is need for Yoruba traditional medicine to be integrated into orthodox medicine. This requires collaboration among relevant institutions for the seamless integration of traditional medicine. Integration of traditional medicines into modern healthcare systems would subject them to appropriate regulation and evidenced-based practice. Integration of TM with Western medicine offers democratized, cheaper, accessible, affordable, and effective health management [27,28].

- *Regulation:* There is need for development of regulation and guidelines for controlling traditional medicines and training of personnel working on traditional medicines.

- *No Central Professional Body:* Although there is a proliferation of Yoruba herbalist associations (such as Yoruba Parapo Traditional Medicine Practitioners Association), there is no central professional body to control their activities, and there is danger of unsubstantiated claim of proficiency in the treatment diseases by herbalists [29].

- *Christian Faith:* Some missionaries condemn the use of traditional medicines and discourage Christians from using them. They also warned their converts against the use of divinations, commonly used in diagnosing diseases. Condemnation of the traditional medicine in its entirety seems excessive and unwarranted [30]. There are some Yoruba Christians who totally avoid any form of traditional medicine believing that prayer is all they need for healing.

- *Complexity:* TM is often perceived as a complex science that stems from a diverse array of traditions, cultures, and worldviews. There is no one-size-fits-all approach. Consult with your doctor before using any TM treatment.

- *No Standards:* Due to absence of standards, a lot of people sell products that are not authentic. This gives the TM industry a bad name. The herbal medicines are generally not adequately researched and are not regulated.

Some of these challenges are shown in Figure 7.8. Other challenges include lack of documentation, poor packaging, and poor sanitation of the environment where drugs are prepared. These challenges must be addressed before the potential of YTM can be fully realized. In spite of the challenges, there is an increasing renewed interest in using the herbs because they have been very useful.

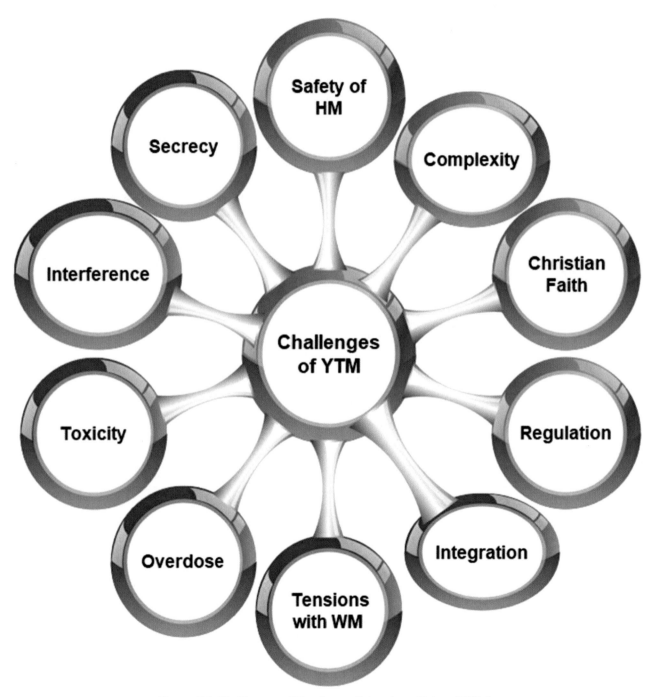

Figure 7.8 Challenges of Yoruba traditional medicine (YTM).

7.8 GLOBALIZATION OF YORUBA MEDICINE

The high cost of Western medical healthcare and the expensive pharmaceutical products have made them unavailable to a majority of people. The Western medicines also have increased side effects and they lack curative treatment for several chronic diseases. They can cure only one-third out of 30,000 human diseases or disorders. As other developing nations, Nigeria is faced with acute shortage of Western-trained doctors and paramedical staff. All this has caused an increasing renewed interest in Yoruba tradition medicine, which is often juxtaposed with modern medicine. The Yoruba tribe stand out when it comes to natural medicines. The YTM is one the various systems of medicinal techniques in the contemporary society. Herbal medicine has survived the modern age and is still a popular practice in Yorubaland. The Yoruba healing systems have attracted the attention of several scholars around the world due to the fact that Yorùbá people are one of the most researched ethno-linguistic groups in Africa [31].

The current trend is the modernization and globalization of Yoruba traditional medicine and products. The WHO has proposed the training of TM practitioners for healthcare services. This will enable the integration of traditional medical systems with national health systems. Thus, the traditional medical practitioners are currently employing some strategies to ensure integration of their practices into the national healthcare delivery. Some professional associations have been formed among traditional healers. These include Yoruba Parapo Traditional Medicine Practitioners Association and National Association of Traditional Medicine Practitioners. These serve as meeting points for healers for social purposes and to share their professional experiences. The Western-trained doctors and government health policy makers should liaison with such associations [31,32].

Yoruba religion has been making its way to the United States, where it is resonating with many Black Americans because it offers them a chance to connect to a spiritual heritage that predates colonization and the transatlantic slave trade. In Brazil, enslaved Yoruba brought their traditions with them. *The Yoruba traditional medicine* is now in high demand in Brazil and in most of the Latin American nations, where they are used for medicinal and spiritual cures. Some age-old Yoruba herbs are known for their efficacy against witchcraft in Brazil.

7.9 CONCLUSION

The Yoruba people are one of the most prominent, urbanized, and cultured peoples on the African continent. They are blessed with natural remedies. According to the World Health Organization, 80% of Africans use traditional medicine for primary healthcare. Traditional healing among the Yoruba people remains a relevant, resilient institution till today in spite of the influence of colonization, westernization, and modernization [33]

Yoruba indigenous medicine has a bright future which can be achieved through collaboration, partnership, and integration with conventional medicine. Some universities in Nigeria have started to offer courses in indigenous African medicines. Africa should continue to seek traditional medicine for home grown solutions to healthcare. Despite fears that some African traditional medicines could be detrimental to health, the number of people patronizing it keeps soaring. More information about Yoruba traditional medicine can be found in books in [34-46] and the following related journals:

- *Journal of Herbal Medicine*
- *Journal of Ethnopharmacology*

- *Yoruba Studies Review*
- *Journal of Traditional Medicine & Clinical Naturopathy*
- *African Journal of Infectious Diseases*
- *African Journal of Traditional, Complementary and Alternative Medicines*
- *East African Medical Journal*
- *International Journal of Traditional and Complementary Medicine*
- *International Journal of Traditional and Natural Medicines*
- *Transactions of the Royal Society of Tropical Medicine & Hygiene* and *International Health*.

REFERENCES

[1] M. N. O. Sadiku, P. O. Adebo, and S. M. Musa, "Traditional Yoruba Medicine: An overview," *International Journal of Trend in Research and Development*, vol. 9, no. 1, January-February 2023, pp. 56-61.

[2] Editorial Board, "Traditional medicine and cure for malaria," May 2018, Unknown Source.

[3] L. C. Saalu, "Nigerian folklore medicinal plants with potential antifertility activity in males: A scientific appraisal," *Research Journal of Medicinal Plants,* vol. 10, 2016, 201-227.

[4] I. A .Paul, "The survival of the Yorùbá healing systems in the modern age," *Yoruba Studies Review,* vol. 2, o. 2, 2018.
https://news.clas.ufl.edu/the-survival-of-the-yoruba-healing-systems-in-the-modern-age/

[5] C. Jorjette, "Yoruba names for herbs and plants – Nigerian medicine,"
https://www.egofelix.com/yoruba-medicine/

[6] "Ifa divination system,"
https://ich.unesco.org/en/RL/ifa-divination-system-00146

[7] "Traditional African medicine and conventional drugs: Friends or enemies?" March 2018,
https://theconversation.com/traditional-african-medicine-and-conventional-drugs-friends-or-enemies-92695

[8] B. O. Ifadamilare, "The science of Yoruba medicine," Unknown Source.

[9] "Herbal medicine 101: How you can harness the power of healing herbs,"
https://www.healthline.com/health/herbal-medicine-101-harness-the-power-of-healing-herbs

[10] V. Awala, "7 Facts about agbo you should know," February 2016,
https://www.informationng.com/2016/02/7-facts-about-agbo-you-should-know.html

[11] C. Muanya, "Ten Nigerian medicinal plants proposed by NMC for standardization,"
https://guardian.ng/features/ten-nigerian-medicinal-plants-proposed-by-nmc-for-standardisation/

[12] J. D. Olowokudejo A. B. Kadiri, and V. A. Travih, "An ethnobotanical survey of herbal markets and medicinal plants in Lagos state of Nigeria," *Ethnobotanical Leaflets,* vol. 2008. Article 116, 2008.

[13] G. O. Adekunle et al., "Cutaneous adornment in the Yoruba of south-western Nigeria – past and present," *International Journal of Dermatology*, vol. 45, no. 1, January 2006, pp.23-27.

[14] S. Anokan, Yoruba Traditional Engagement List: Bride price list fro grooms-to-be,"
https://naijaglamwedding.com/yoruba-engagement-list/

[15] "The dangers of drinking agbo jedi jedi and other 'Yoruba' herbal medicine,"
http://ng.dailyadvent.com/others/2019/03/20/the-dangers-of-drinking-agbo-jedi-jedi-and-other-yoruba-herbal-medicine/

[16] "Traditional African medicine," *Wikipedia,* the free encyclopedia
https://en.wikipedia.org/wiki/Traditional_African_medicine

[17] "The cure for malaria could be in your backyard,"
https://ctegd.uga.edu/the-cure-for-malaria-could-be-in-your-backyard/

[18] C. Muanya, "Herbal 'cures' for multi-drug resistant typhoid fever,"
https://guardian.ng/features/health/herbal-cures-for-multi-drug-resistant-typhoid-fever/#:~:text
=Neem%20tree-,SeveralL%20studies%20have%20identified%20plants%20that%20could%20be%
20effectively%20used,(pawpaw)%20and%20Morinda%20lucida.

[19] "10 Yoruba herbs for erectile dysfunction,"
https://nigerianfinder.com/yoruba-herbs-for-erectile-dysfunction/#

[20] "10 Herbs that may help lower high blood pressure,"
https://www.healthline.com/nutrition/herbs-to-lower-blood-pressure

[21] B. Okpara, "18 Medicinal plants/herbs for treating diarrhea," March 2016,
https://globalfoodbook.com/18-medicinal-plants-herbs-for-treating-diarrhea

[22] U. Eshemokha, "Nigeria herbs for treating diabetes including Yoruba herbs for diabetes," June 2020,
https://nimedhealth.com.ng/2020/06/16/nigerian-herbs-for-treating-diabetes-including-yoruba-
herbs-for-diabetes/

[23] S. Rashmi and S. Shilpy "Herbs and botanical ingredients with beneficial effects on blood sugar
levels in pre-diabetes," *Herbal Medicine,* vol. 2, no. 1, February 2016.

[24] "How traditional medicine transformed my life – Ooni Of Ife," September 2020,
https://www.vanguardngr.com/2020/09/how-traditional-medicine-transformed-my-life-ooni-of-ife/

[25] W. Koster-Oyekan, "Infertility among Yoruba women: Perceptions on causes, treatments and
consequences," *African Journal of Reproductive Health,* vol. 3, no. 1, 1999, pp. 13-26.

[26] "Benefits of herbal medicine," *Proceedings of the 2nd International Conference on Herbal & Traditional
Medicine,* June 20-21, 2019, Dubai, UAE, |https://www.omicsonline.org/conferences-list/
benefits-of-herbal-medicine

[27] I. A. Oreagba, K. A. Oshikoya, and M. Amachree, "Herbal medicine use among urban residents
in Lagos, Nigeria," *BMC Complementary and Alternative Medicine,* vol. 11, 2011.

[28] C. Jansen et al., "Medicine in motion: Opportunities, challenges and data analytics-based solutions
for traditional medicine integration into western medical practice," *Journal of Ethnopharmacology,*
vol. 267, March 2021.

[29] T. R. Oyelakin, "Yoruba traditional medicine and the challenge of integration." *Journal of Pan
African Studies,* vol. 3, no. 3, September 2009,

[30] D. D. O. Oyebola, "Professional associations, ethics and discipline among Yoruba traditional healers
of Nigeria," *Social Science & Medicine. Part B: Medical Anthropology,* vol. 15, no. 2, April 1981, pp. 87-92.

[31] "The survival of the Yorùbá healing systems in the modern age,"
https://news.clas.ufl.edu/the-survival-of-the-yoruba-healing-systems-in-the-modern-age/

[32] O. Awodele et al., "Towards integrating traditional medicine (TM) into National Health Care
Scheme (NHCS): Assessment of TM practitioners' disposition in Lagos," *Journal of Herbal Medicine,*
2011, pp. 90-94.

[33] S. B. Amusa and C. A. Ogidan, "Yoruba Indigenous medical knowledge: A study of the nature,
dynamisms, and resilience of Yoruba medicine," *Journal of the Knowledge Economy,* vol. 8, no. 3,
September 2017, pp. 977-986.

[34] L. Omotosho and O. Odejobi, *Computational Ontology Model: Yoruba Traditional Medicine Perspective.* LAP LAMBERT Academic Publishing, 2021.

[35] N. S. Lawal, M. N. O. Sadiku, and P. A. Dopamu, *Understanding Yoruba Life and Culture.* African World Press, 2004.

[36] M. M. Iwu, *Handbook of African Medicinal Plants.* Boca Raton, FL: CRC Press; 2nd edition, 2014.

[37] D. O. Oyebola, *African Traditional Medicine: Practices Among the Yoruba of Nigeria.* Christian Faith Publishing, 2020.

[38] M. O. Adekson, *The Yoruba Traditional Healers of Nigeria.* Routledge, 2012.

[39] T. M. Sawandi, *African Medicine: A Complete Guide to Yoruba Healing Science and African Herbal Remedies.* CreateSpace Independent Publishing Platform, 2nd edition, 2017.

[40] A. D. Buckley, *Yoruba Medicine.* Athelia Henrietta Press, 1997.

[41] A. Adodo and, M. M. Iwu, *Healing Plants of Nigeria: Ethnomedicine and Therapeutic Applications (Traditional Herbal Medicines for Modern Times).* Boca Raton, FL: CRC Press, 2020.

[42] O. Olagunju, *Therapeutic Practices in Yoruba Traditional Religions.* KS OmniScriptum Publishing, 2012.

[43] E. A. Oke and B. E. Owumi, *Reading in Medical Sociology.* Ibadan, Nigeria: Resource Development and Management Services, 1996.

[44] J. DeJong, *Traditional Medicine in Sub-Saharan Africa: Its Importance And Potential Policy Options.* The World Bank, 1991.

[45] T. Falola and M. M. Heaton (eds.), *Traditional and Modern Health Systems in Nigeria.* Trenton, NJ: Africa World Press, 2006.

[46] J. I. Durodola, *Scientific Insights into Yoruba Traditional Medicine.* New York: Trado–Medical Books, 1986.

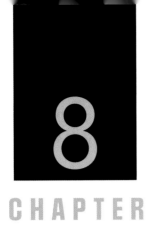

CHAPTER

Persian Traditional Medicine

"Wherever the art of medicine is loved, there is also a love of humanity." - Anonymous

8.1 INTRODUCTION

Since time immemorial, human beings have tried to create means of survival and protection against all poisons and illnesses. They were motivated by the universal desire for longevity. Since the beginning of civilization, herbal, animal, and mineral medicaments have been used to treat diseases. The practice of traditional medicine is deeply rooted in the cultural heritage of an ethic group. It constitutes an integral part of the culture of the indigenous people. According to the World Health Organization, traditional herbal medicines are naturally occurring, with minimal or no industrial processing that have been used to treat illness. Traditional herbal medicines are getting significant attention in global health debates.

Iran is formerly known as Persia. Iranian traditional medicine (also known as Persian medicine or Tebb e Sonnati) is one of famous forms of traditional medicine. It is also one of the most ancient forms of medicine in the world, with more than 4000 years of history, consists of the sum total of all the knowledge and practices used in diagnosis, prevention, and treatment in Iran from ancient times to the present. Persian traditional medicines (PTM) may be regarded as the sum total of all the knowledge and practices of medicine used in Persia from ancient times till today. The medicines have been used and proven for over centuries and have been recommended from ancient times. They give more attention and importance to the prevention of disease rather than its cure [1].

Iran is located in southwest Asia. It is a country of mountains and deserts. It is regarded as the jewel in Islam's crown. The nation consists of numerous ethnic groups. Although many languages originated from Iran, Persian is the most used language. Persian is considered the language of intellectuals during much of the 2nd millennium.

The first medical center was established in Persia (Iran) in the 6th century.

This chapter provides an introduction to Persian traditional medicine (PTM) in Iran. It begins by providing some historical background on PTM. It describes the concept of PTM. It discusses some Persian herbal medicines. It gives some typical applications of PTM. It highlights some benefits and challenges of PTM. It covers the globalization of PTM. The last section concludes with comments.

8.2 BRIEF HISTORY OF PERSIAN MEDICINE

A brief historical background may be necessary in order to appreciate the significance of Persian traditional medicine. Studies show that earliest records of the history of ancient Iranian medicine can be found in 8,000 to 6,500 B.C. Iranians believe that food is medicine and every disease starts in the gut. The practice of medicine in Persia has a long and prolific history.

The Iranian medicine was combined by different medical traditions from Mesopotamia, Egypt, India, China, and Greece for more than 4000 years. Medical sciences has a long history in Middle and Near East and goes back to the ancient Mesopotamian period.

A medicine center was found at Gondi Sapur University in the 4th century AD, in which the first international medicine congress was held. The practice of Iranian medicine was interrupted by the Arab invasion (630 AD). However, the advances of the Sassanid period were continued and expanded. The Sassanid Empire in Persia (224–637 AD) ruled one of the most influential eras in world history. Medicine was well organized in the official Sassanid system. Globally, medicine reached its peak with the rise of Islam in Iran. The conquest of Islam in 7th century improved trade and boasted book publishing. After the Prophet Muhammad's death in 632, Islam expands beyond Arabia to Persia, Palestine, Syria, Lebanon, Iraq, and North Africa. In Baghdad, the celebrated Iranian physician and philosopher, Abu Ali Sina (980-1037), known as Avicenna in the west, wrote 100 books on many subjects. His most famous compendium, *The Canon of Medicine,* a five-volume work encompassing all known medical knowledge of the time, was the final authority on medical matters in Europe for several centuries [2].

Following the establishment of the Tehran university school of medicine in 1934 and the return of Iranian graduates from the medical schools in Europe, much progress was made in the development and availability of trained manpower in medicine. After the Islamic revolution and establishment of Islamic Republic of Iran by late Imam Khomeini in 1979, all the foreign doctors in rural clinics were replaced by young Iranian medical graduates [3].

8.3 CONCEPT OF PERSIAN TRADITIONAL MEDICINE

Iranian traditional medicine strongly focuses on prioritizing health maintenance and disease prevention over treatment. It is based on four basic substances, called humors, that divide human fluid into four basic types: Blood (Dam), Phlegm (Balgham), Yellow bile (Ṣafrā'), and Black bile (Saudā'). They are illustrated in Figure 8.1 and explained as follows [4]:

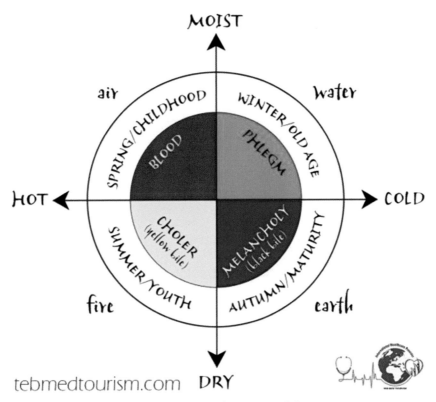

Figure 8.1 Four basic types [4].

- *Blood:* This is the most abundant and the most important humor in the body which will be formed by eating food. Children in particular need larger amounts of "blood" for growth and they get it by consuming foodstuff.
- *Phlegm:* Next to blood, phlegm is the second most abundant humor in the body. It is a slimy liquid very much like water (colorless, odorless, and tasteless) and it can be found in body parts. Phlegm can be considered as a kind of food supply for the body.
- *Yellow bile:* This acts as a diluent and facilitates the transfer of blood and nutrients from capillaries to the remote body organs. It is also in charge of metabolism of fats and digestion. Yellow bile is tasked with cleaning up the digestive system, vascular tissues, and genitalia.
- *Black bile:* This strengthens body parts. It is sparse but essential to the body. The right amounts of black bile keep bones healthy and strong. Bones, teeth, and tendons primarily live off black bile. Lack of black bile in the body will compromise bone's strength and the tendons function.

When the four humors are in balance, they bring physical and mental health. Any excess or deficiency of any of the four bodily fluids in a person may lead to diseases and disabilities The basic knowledge of four senses of humor as a healing system was developed by Hakim Ibn Sina in his medical encyclopedia *The Canon of Medicine.* The old medical system is a tradition with roots further in the ancient Iranian and Indian past.

Persian traditional medicine determines hotness (*Garmi*) and coldness (*Sardi*) of foods by the impact that they have on the human body. Hot foods are usually eaten during cold weathers to keep the body warm. Cold foods are consumed during the warm seasons. They are harder to digest and harder to assimilate. Determining which foods are appropriate for your temperament is crucial to maintaining sound health and wellbeing.

Persian traditional medicine (PTM) is a holistic medicine that prioritizes health maintenance over treating diseases. It provides great attention to the spiritual aspects of life as well as somatic aspects to maintain human health. Nutrition plays a crucial role in maintaining body health. The quality and quantity of foods would influence mental health. Therefore, the traditional physician should correct the nutritional habit of the patients as the first step toward healing.

The lifestyle rules in PTM focus on six fundamental and guiding principles, known as *Setah Zaroriah* in Persian [5]:

- Nutrition
- Environment
- Physical activity
- Sleeping patterns
- Emotions
- Ridding the body of waste materials

These principles are illustrated in Figure 8.2 [6]. One must take these basic principles into account in maintaining sound health. Learning about the daily lifestyle of the patients, their family and social interactions and health, their sleep patterns, and daily habits can provide important information that helps uncover their health condition.

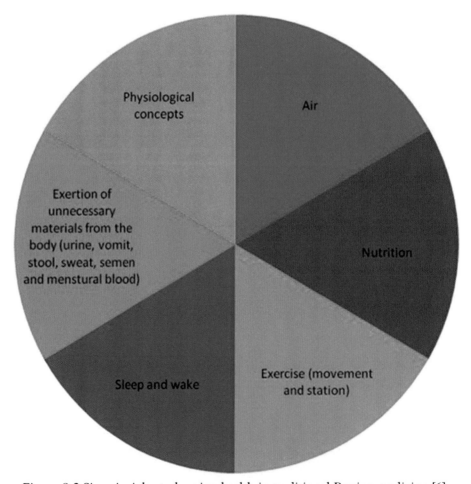

Figure 8.2 Six principles to keeping health in traditional Persian medicine [6].

8.4 IRANIAN HERBS

Medicinal plants have been widely used by people all over the world. Herbal medicine, also known as herbalism, is based on the use of plants for healing and the maintenance of health. It is often used after medical examinations and diagnosis have been done. They are based on their effectiveness, efficacy, and properties, to eliminate the symptoms of the disease.

Medicinal plants have attracted the attention of Iranians from ancient times. Over the years different kinds of extraction and preparing herbal medicines were developed and used. There are 8100 plant species and about 2300 aromatic spices in Iran now. Some of these herbal medicines are used all over the world. Herbal remedies are consumed in many forms, including teas, tisanes (or infusions), decoctions, macerations, tinctures, and elixirs. Different kinds of diseases are cured by means of herbal therapy. Figure 8.3 displays various types of Persian traditional medicines [7]. Persian traditional practitioners can use these traditional medicines to cure diseases.

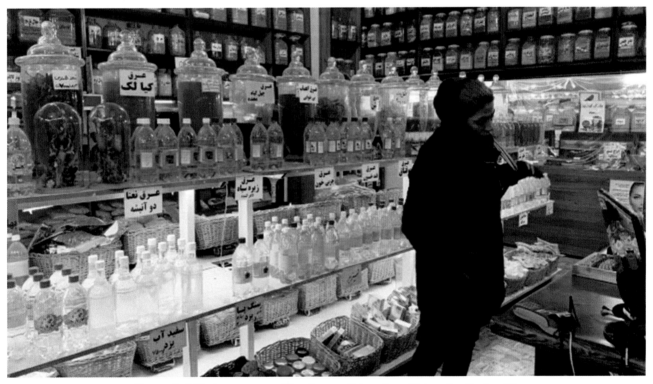

Figure 8.3 Various types of Persian traditional medicines in display [7].

Figure 8.4 shows Mostafa Rahemi, a Persian traditional medicine man who heals using herbs and plants [8]. Some of these herbal medicines are produced commercially these days. For example, Figure 8.5 shows medicinal herbs effective for gray hair [9].

The most common herbal medicines among Iranians are [10–12]:

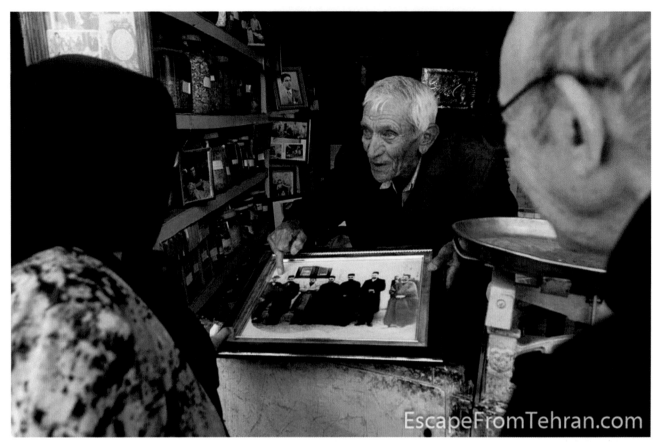

Figure 8.4 Mostafa Rahemi, the Persian traditional medicine man [8].

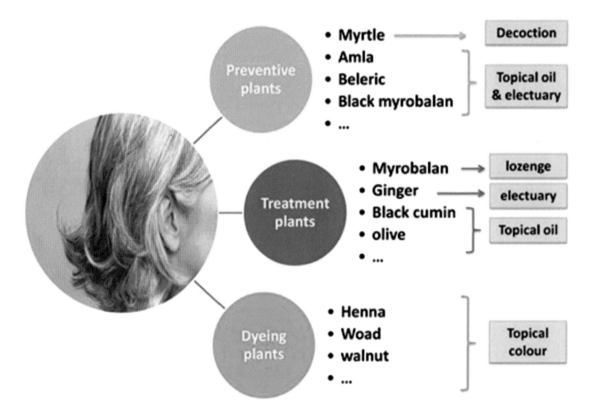

Figure 8.5 Medicinal herbs effective for gray hair [9].

- *Borage* (golgavezaban): It grows in the northern parts of Iran and its purple flower is using in the same way that tea leaves are using.
- *Shahla is* continuing an Iranian tradition of medicine going back several thousand years.
- *Valerian* (Sonboletip): Valerian is one of those Persian herbal medicine mostly using to calm down the nerves. It is shown in Figure 8.6 [13]. It is useful for those who suffer from insomnia.

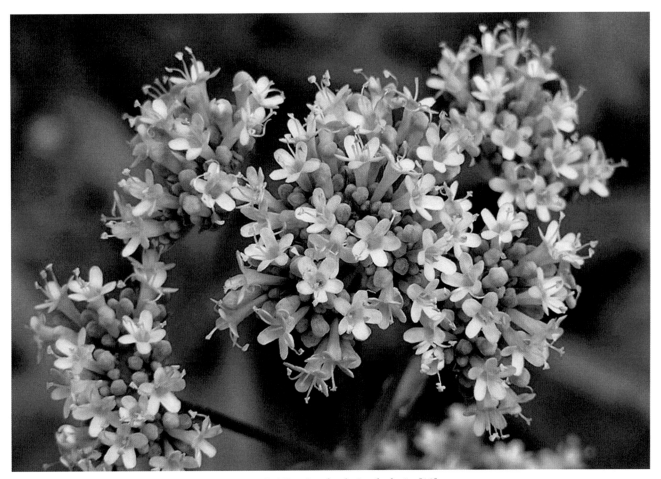

Figure 8.6 Persian herb Sonboletip [13].

- *Rocket seeds* (khakeshir): These tiny brown seeds have great health benefits. Khakshir is a natural liver detoxifier. It also improves skin and clears the blemishes.
- *Chicory* (kasni): This has some advantages such as cooling nature to reduce the body temperature and it is also good for liver diseases.
- *Thyme* (Avishan): This herbal tea is good for a dry cough and upper respiratory tract inflammation as it is a kind of disinfectant. It is also good for digestion and sleeping problems.
- *Badranjboye* (dragonhead): This Persian herb helps address difficulty sleeping. Drinking dragonhead herbal tea (an hour before going to sleep) can help respond to sleep problems. The dragonhead is from mint family and has calming effects.
- *Oils* are one of the most ancient forms of natural herbal medicines. Administration of herbal oils is rooted in traditional knowledge. Medicinal oils have been used to target particular areas of the body to combat specific ailments.

125

- *Althaea* (Marshmallow): This has been under consumption over the past few centuries to manage various diseases. It has been used for the treatment of dry cough, fever, inflammation, constipation, as well as burns in children and adults.

8.5 APPLICATIONS OF PERSIAN TRADITIONAL MEDICINE

Persian traditional medicine has been applied successfully to treat various diseases such as coughing, constipation, premature ovarian failure, neurological diseases, sleeplessness, liver diseases, psychiatry diseases, infertility, impotence, and erectile dysfunction. The main goal is to correctly diagnose the disease and to treat the patients in the shortest time. The traditional medicine has been successful in treating various diseases including neurological diseases, psychiatry diseases, women diseases, liver cleansing, and infertility.

- *Constipation*: There is no effective modern drug for constipation. However, there are many medicinal material in Persian traditional medicine that can be used for treatment of constipation. Constipation is one of the most harmful factors in cardiac health. Four important medicines with laxative effect are Prunus domestica, ficus cariaca, Cassia fistula, and Cucurbita maxima [14].
- *Headache:* This is one of the most common public health problems in the world. Migraine is the second most common cause of headaches after tension headaches. The symptoms of migraine include nausea, sensitivity to light, and decrease in productivity. Effective drugs are required to treat headache. The combination of Viola odorata, Rosa damascene, and Coriandrum sativum have been found to be effective in treating patients with migraine headache [15].
- *Depression:* This is one of the most common mental disorders around the world. Depression and loneliness are important factors that endanger the health of people, especially the elderly. Traditional Persian medicine has provided remedies for depression management. Taken together, apigenin, caffeic acid, catechin, chlorogenic acid, citral, ellagic acid, esculetin, ferulic acid, gallic acid, gentiopicroside, hyperoside, kaempferol, limonene, linalool, lycopene, naringin, protocatechuic acid, quercetin, resveratrol, rosmarinic acid, and umbelliferone are suitable for the management of depression [16].
- *Sleeplessness:* Sleep is physical, passive, and mental rest. Sleeplessness or insomnia is a sleep disorder which affects almost half of the general population. Iranian traditional herbal remedies can be used to address the problem of sleeplessness. Drinking dragonhead herbal tea can help with difficulty in sleeping. This tea is from mint family. Five grams of the tea in hot water in a mug, taken an hour before sleep, will produce calming effects [17].
- *Liver Cleansing:* Liver is one of the most important organs in the body. It is one of the three commanders in the body (brain, heart, liver) that manages nutrition and growth. It must be protected by cleansing and detoxifying it using effective herbal medicines. Such cleansing is in favor of health and vitality. Persian traditional medicine is one of the best and safest methods for liver cleansing. Artichoke stimulates bile secretion and helps eliminate toxins accumulated in the liver. Turmeric tea is an important method of detoxifying the liver. Fresh turmeric, fresh ginger, black pepper, cinnamon, coconut milk, and honey are often used to make turmeric tea. The tea should be used in the form of tea for 45 days (during the day after meals) in order to regulate liver enzymes [18,19].

- *COVID-19:* This is a life-threatening viral infection. The disease is spreading fast, and needs to be prevented from spreading. The World Health Organization (WHO) and medical experts from all over the world consider the only way to fight and prevent the Coronavirus is regular hand washing and home quarantine. Everything that is used is based on try and error. When the modern medical system cannot treat COVID-19, the traditional medical community has explored its remedy by herbal medicines. As the new corona virus progresses, the death toll continues to increase, and this poses a major threat to the world. Professor Khairandish known as the "Father of Iranian Traditional Medicine" treated the virus that the world's medical science has nothing to offer. His current success in treating the corona patients saved countless lives [20-22].

- *Cardiovascular Diseases:* These are major health complications. The management of heart diseases as a prevention step or as treatment with low-cost procedures like lifestyle modifications are important current trends. One of the most important strategies for reducing these consequences is to correct unhealthy family diets. Choosing right, effective foods based on individual temperament is recommended by Persian physicians. Besides the foods effective in retaining health for cardiac patients, saffron has a special role [6]. The concept of nutrition in heart diseases has had a successful background at least from 1000 years ago in Persia.

- *Erectile Dysfunction:* Due to health, cultural, and individual differences, the global prevalence of ED differs from one nation to another. The high costs of its conventional treatment has motivated researchers to look for alternative approaches to the treatment of sexual dysfunction. The use of medicinal plants for male reproductive function is associated with their antioxidant activity, since they present in their compositions phytochemical compounds able to inhibit spermatic membrane lipid peroxidation. Various medicinal herbs have been used for impotency and erectile dysfunction [23].

- *Epilepsy:* This is an important issue in in the field of neuroscience. It is a disease prevalent on a global scale. In Iranian traditional medicine, herbal remedies have been used for centuries to treat seizures. Iranian scientists such as Ibn Sina and Rhazes have defined epilepsy, described its signs and symptoms, and gave different approaches to prevent and treat it. Twenty-five plants have been identified as herbal remedies to treat epilepsy. Currently, the five most important herbals in Iranian traditional medicine for treating epilepsy are Canon, al-Hawi, al-Abniah 'an Haqaeq al Adwia, Tuhfat al-Mu'minin, and Makhzan ul-Adwia. These herbs have been pharmacologically investigated for their antiepileptic activity and have shown anticonvulsant properties [24].

- *Infertility:* This is the inability to conceive after sexual intercourse. Current treatments for male infertility are expensive with low successful rates. *Withania somnifera* is a medicinal plant that can be used in medicinal treatments. Its extract is widely used herbal medicines for treating infertility and sexual dysfunction. The plant is known for its potential to promote health and longevity by preventing the aging process and revitalizing the body in debilitated conditions [25].

- *Obesity:* Diabetes mellitus is the most common endocrine disorder and a leading cause of morbidity and mortality. It is a major risk factor for many diseases, especially in children. Obesity is a major risk factor for diabetes, cardiovascular diseases, cancer, depression, and other diseases. Iran was one of the seven countries having the highest prevalence of childhood obesity. Paying more attention to the prevention of obesity is better than its cure. Unhealthy lifestyle such as irregular sleep, overeating, lack of exercise plays an important role in obesity. For example, nutrition has a crucial role in maintaining body health and overeating may cause accumulation of unhealthy substances in the body. PTM treatment of obesity requires observing the six essential principles in management of pediatric obesity. These factors are: air, food and drink, sleep and wakefulness, evacuation and retention, body movement, mental movement and repose. PTM emphasizes physical therapy in the treatment of obesity [26].

- *Cancer:* This is a major public health problem and is the second leading cause of death with profound socio-economic consequences worldwide. Many patients with cancer want to do everything to fight the disease, manage its symptoms, and cope with the side effects of treatment. Conventional treatment of cancer are chemotherapy, radiation, and surgery. Cancer patients often use traditional health approaches, such as nutritional supplements, special diets, herbal medicine, acupuncture, massage, and yoga. This healing approach takes account of the whole person, including all aspects of lifestyle of life for patients. Eating fruit, vegetables, whole grains, and beans will lower the risk of developing cancer [27,28].

- *Ageing:* Old age is an important period of life in human beings and should not be regarded as a disease The Persians often says, "Old age may be considered the longest period of life." Age increase is associated with higher prevalence of cognitive disorders including forgetfulness, dementia, Xerostomia, and osteoarthritis of the knee. These are common problems in an elderly population, with a range of causes that affect important aspects of life, such as chewing, swallowing, and speaking. Memory injury is the most major factor in these conditions. With increase of world population age, Alzheimer's disease dementia is becoming more prevalent. Osteoarthritis of the knee is one of the main complications with chronic pain and locomotor disability that most elderly populations all around the world suffer from. Traditional Persian medicine has given more attention and importance to the prevention of diseases rather than their cure. A regular moderate physical activity to maintain the stamina of the elderly, healthy diet, and good relationship with family and friends should always be considered for the elderly. The Persian medicine involves the administration of compound medicines comprising numerous medicinal herbs [29].

Other diseases that have been treated by PTM include premature ovarian failure, ulcerative colitis, impotence, dry mouth, measles, menopause, ulcers, urinalysis, wound healing, dementia, dermatitis, coughing, asthma, and oral diseases (such as tooth loss, periodontal disease, and dental caries)

8.6 BENEFITS

There is a growing interest in the use of Persian medicines. A significant amount of people in developing nations presently use herbal medicine for primary healthcare. The base of PTM is prevention from illness. As a result, several remedies have been recommended for staying healthy. The major benefits of PTM include the following:

- *Holistic Medicine:* Persian traditional medicine is a holistic medicine which has been based on individual differences. Everybody has a definite Mizaj which determines all physical or mental characteristics. Persian medicine provides great attention to the spiritual aspects of life as well as somatic aspects to maintain human health. People will not just eat and drink for pleasure, they will maintain a good life, physical health, and spiritual satisfaction.

- *Preventive Medicine:* These days, preventive medicine is neglected in medical conception. As Desiderius Erasmus well said, "Prevention is better than cure!" Persian traditional medicine is based on preventive healthcare. Its strength comes from prioritizing health maintenance over treating diseases.
- *Readily Available:* Persian herbs are available absolutely everywhere from restaurants to grocery stores. They are readily available at Attâri, which are traditional stores in any street where you can find all kinds of medicinal herbs, spices, natural soaps, oil, and shampoos. All Attaris are required to display their license because they must never sell counterfeit or addictive drugs.

8.7 CHALLENGES

Persian traditional medicine has been overshadowed by the Western medicine over the past two centuries. Some medicinal trees mentioned in classical texts of Persian traditional herbal medicine do no longer grow in Iran today. Many modern doctors are skeptical about the impact of herbal therapy in the management of various diseases.

8.8 GLOBALIZATION OF PERSIAN MEDICINE

Persian traditional medicines (PTM) have been used for centuries and their effects have been proven over the years. Traditional medicine has grown significantly in recent years in Iran. Iran exports 1,450 tons herbal medicine. Many patients in developing and developed countries have turned to traditional therapies for treating their illnesses. This is due to the cost; modern medicines are prohibitively expensive in those nations.

WHO declared that Persian traditional medicine has the potential to gain international recognition and WHO must support its globalization. This will introduce its capacities to the world [30].

Today the Islamic Republic of Iran is moving towards sharing its useful medical treasures with mankind all over the world and to participate in integrative medicine. The Ministry of Health in Iran has an office for traditional medicine. Courses on traditional medicine are offered in the main medical universities. Every clinical service using the traditional remedies must be certified by the Ministry of Health. The School of Persian Medicine, shown in Figure 8.7, is the first and most distinguished Persian traditional medicine in the Middle East [31]. It promotes traditional medicine and encourages developing new medicine thorough research.

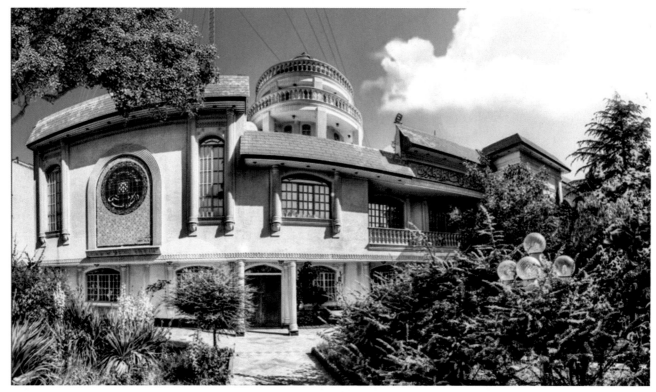

Figure 8.7 School of Persian Medicine [31].

8.9 CONCLUSION

Persian traditional medicine is a set of knowledge and skills in the diagnosis, prevention, and treatment of diseases from ancient times till now. Iranians have always relied on their traditional medicines to treat various diseases. The development and promotion of traditional medicine around the world constitute honor and respect to the culture and heritage of the people everywhere. There is a growing tendency towards traditional medicine in the world as well as growing interest in Persian Medicine in Iran. Considering the importance and richness of traditional Iranian medicine, Persian traditional medicine needs revival. More information about Persian traditional medicine can be found in the books in [32–38] and related journals:

- *Archives of Iranian Medicine*
- *Iranian Journal of Public Health*
- *Iranian Journal of Medical Sciences*
- *Journal of Integrative Medicine*
- *Journal of Medicinal Plants Research*
- *Journal of Traditional and Complementary Medicine*
- *Journal of Islamic and Iranian Traditional Medicine*
- *Current Traditional Medicine*
- *Traditional Medicine Research*
- *Traditional and Integrative Medicine*

REFERENCES

[1]   M. N. O. Sadiku, U. C. Chukwu, A. Ajayi-Majebi, S. M. Musa, "Persian traditional medicine: An introduction," *International Journal of Trend in Scientific Research and Development*, vol. 6, no. 1, November-December 2021, pp.1020-1021.

[2]   "History of ancient medicine in Iran," http://drjafargholi.com/en/history-of-ancient-medicine-in-iran/

[3]   J. Pourahmad, "History of medical sciences in Iran," *Iranian Journal of Pharmaceutical Research,* vol. 7, no. 2, 2008, pp. 93-99.

[4]   "Iranian traditional medicine," https://tebmedtourism.com/iranian-traditional-medicine/

[5]   "East meets West in medicine," May 2021, https://www.sharp.com/health-news/east-meets-west-in-medicine.cfm

[5]   G. Kordafshari, H. M. Kenari, and M. M. Esfahani, "Nutritional aspects to prevent heart diseases in traditional Persian medicine," *Journal of Evidence-Based Integrative Medicine*, October 2014.

[7]   "Rise in Iranian traditional medicine as Covid crisis grows," https://www.ft.com/content/8c1ce774-c0af-4f48-b585-4edb92e12ad9

[8]   A. Torkzadeh, "The last medicine man," March 2017, https://medium.com/escapefromtehran/the-last-medicine-man-a1fbce0f61f8

[9]   M. Raeiszadeh, M. Rameshk, and S. K.i Khandani, "Medicinal herbs effective for gray hair in traditional Persian medicine," *Current Traditional Medicine*, vol. 7, no. 3, 2021.

[10]   "Persian herbal medicine," https://www.irandestination.com/persian-herbal-medicine/

[11]   A. Hamedi et al., "Herbal medicinal oils in traditional Persian medicine," *Pharmaceutical Biology*, vol. 51, no. 9, 2013, pp. 1208-1218.

[12]   "6 Common Iranian home remedies you should know," February 2019, https://www.mypersiancorner.com/6-common-iranian-home-remedies/

[13]   "Persian herbal medicine," https://www.irandestination.com/persian-herbal-medicine/

[14]   S. A. Mozaffarpur et al., "Introduction of natural medicinal material effective in treatment of constipation in Persian traditional medicine," *Medical History,* vol. 3, no. 9, July 2012, pp. 79-95.

[15]   M. Kamali et al., "The effectiveness of combination of Viola odorata L., Rosa damascena mill and coriandrum sativum L. on quality of life of patients with migraine headaches: A randomized, double blinded, placebo - controlled clinical," *Traditional and Integrative Medicine,* vol. 4, no. 4, 2019, pp. 181-190.

[16]   A. Jalali, N. Firouzabadi, M. M. Zarshenas, "Pharmacogenetic-based management of depression: Role of traditional Persian medicine," *Phytotheraphy Research,* vol. 25, no. 9, September 2021, pp. 5031-5052.

[17]   S. M. Mirghazanfari, "Can't sleep? Persian medicine helps address difficulty sleeping," July 2018 https://www.tehrantimes.com/news/425706/Can-t-sleep-Persian-medicine-helps-address-difficulty-sleeping

[18]   "Traditional herbal medicine for liver cleansing," https://www.google.com/search?q=Traditional+Herbal+Medicine+for+Liver+Cleansing&rlz=1C1CHBF_enUS910US910&oq=Traditional+Herbal+Medicine+for+Liver+Cleansing&aqs=chrome..69i57.2445j0j7&sourceid=chrome&ie=UTF-8

[19] A. Zarei, S. Noroozi, and E. Khadem, "A review on the structure and function of liver from Avicenna point of view and its comparison with conventional medicine," *Traditional and Integrative Medicine,* vol. 4, no. 1, 2019, pp. 28–36.

[20] M. Johnston, "What is the role of ITM in health and well-being?" https://zenithoffacts.quora.com/What-is-the-role-of-ITM-in-health-and-well-being-Iranian-traditional-medicine-ITM-https-virtualengineering-tech-I

[21] M. Jafari, "Cholera was stronger than corona, and we treated it," June 2020, https://www.linkedin.com/pulse/cholera-stronger-than-corona-we-treated-dr-may-jafari-phd

[22] M. B. Siahpoosh, "How can Persian medicine (traditional Iranian medicine) be effective to control COVID-19?" *Traditional and Integrative Medicine,* vol. 5, no. 2, 2020, pp. 46-48.

[23] M. Nimrouzi, A. M. Jaladat, M. M. Zarshenas, "A panoramic view of medicinal plants traditionally applied for impotence and erectile dysfunction in Persian medicine," *Journal of Traditional and Complementary Medicine,* vol. 10, no. 1, January 2020, pp. 7-12.

[24] S. Sahranavard, S. Ghafari, and M. Mosaddegh, "Medicinal plants used in Iranian traditional medicine to treat epilepsy," *Seizure,* vol. 23, no. 5, May 2014, pp. 328-332.

[25] M. Y. P. Teixeira and C. O. D. de Araujo, "Effect of Withania somnifera in the treatment of male infertility: A literature review," *Journal of Medicinal Plants Research,* vol. 13, no. 18, November 2019, pp. 473-479.

[26] L. Hamidnia et al., "Life style management of pediatric obesity based on traditional Persian medicine: a narrative review," *International Journal of Pediatrics,* vol. 6, no. 6, 2018, pp. 7759-7768.

[27] G. Heydarirad and H. Rezaeizadeh, "An evidence based approach to integrative oncology (traditional herbal remedies and complementary medicine) for the management of complications in head and neck cancers," http://www.smgebooks.com/head-neck-cancer/chapters/HNC-16-03.pdf

[28] B. Javadi, "Diet therapy for cancer prevention and treatment based on traditional Persian medicine," *Nutrition and Cancer,* vol. 70, no. 3, 2018, pp. 376-403.

[29] M. M. Parvizi et al., "Health recommendations for the elderly in the viewpoint of traditional Persian medicine," *Shiraz E-Medical Journal,* vol. 9, no. 1, 2018.

[30] " Iranian traditional medicine can expand globally: WHO," January 2019, https://www.tehrantimes.com/news/432457/Iranian-traditional-medicine-can-expand-globally-WHO

[31] "School of Persian Medicine," http://en.tums.ac.ir/en/content/238/school-of-persian-medicine

[32] S. Angha, *Tebb e Sonnati e Iran (The Traditional Medicine of Iran).* M.T.O. Shahmaghsoudi Printing Center, 1984.

[33] A. A. Minaeifar, K. Bamdad, and S. Dehghani, *Some Common Herbs In Iranian Traditional Medicine.* LAP LAMBERT Academic Publishing, 2018.

[34] H. Ebrahimnejad, *Medicine in Iran: Profession, Practice and Politics, 1800-1925.* Palgrave MacMillan US 2015.

[35] M. Shirzad et al., *Iranian Traditional Medicine: A Dictionary (Arabic-Persian-English).* Traditional Medicine and Materia Medica Research Center, 2014.

[36] J. Hunter, *Herbal Medicinal Oils in Traditional Persian Medicine.* Boston, MA: Medicare Health Science, 2022.

[37] M. Naseri and M. Parviz, *Maintaining Health in the View Point of Persian Medicine.* LAP LAMBERT Academic Publishing, 2nd edition, 2019.

[38] M. Reza, T. Saberi, and Z. Sinaei, *Iranian Traditional Medicine: A Dictionary (Arabic-Persian-English).* Moein Publications, 2016.

CHAPTER

Traditional Arabic and Islamic Medicine

"Make use of medical treatment, for Allah has not made a disease without appointing a remedy for it, with the exception of one disease: old age." -- Prophet Muhammad

9.1 INTRODUCTION

Health and disease are vitally important to rich and poor alike. From the beginning of time, man has relied on natural products, such as plants, animals, microorganisms, and marine organisms, in medicines to alleviate and treat diseases. The traditional Chinese medicine have flourished for hundreds of years. Arab and Muslim scholars introduced hundreds of natural products, which include plants and animal products mentioned in the Holy Quran and in the Prophetic tradition. Natural products can broadly be classified into three groups: Herbal-based, animal-based, or mineral-based products. The treatment of human ailments by using medicines derived from animals is known as zootherapy [1].

Traditional medicine is very popular among the population around the world, especially in the Arab region. From the founding of Islam in the 6th century, the Arabic world became the center of medical knowledge. Islamic medicine built upon the legacies of Greek and Roman physicians and scholars such as Hippocrates.

Medicine was part of medieval Islamic culture. The achievements in medieval Islamic medicine were groundbreaking. The medieval Islamic world produced some of the greatest medical thinkers in history. Medieval Islamic medicine improved understanding of the body's functions, established hospitals, developed medical knowledge, translated medical texts into Arabic, and the incorporated female doctors. Medieval Islamic doctors developed new techniques in medicine, dissection, surgery, and pharmacology. They performed more surgeries than their Greek and Roman predecessors [2]. Medieval Islamic medications were usually plant-based and largely depended on herbs and superstition [3]. Figure 9.1 shows special tools used by medieval surgeons [4]. In the Middle Ages, some women from the families of famous physicians received elite medical training. Such wise woman would provide potions, typically shown in Figure 9. 2 [4].

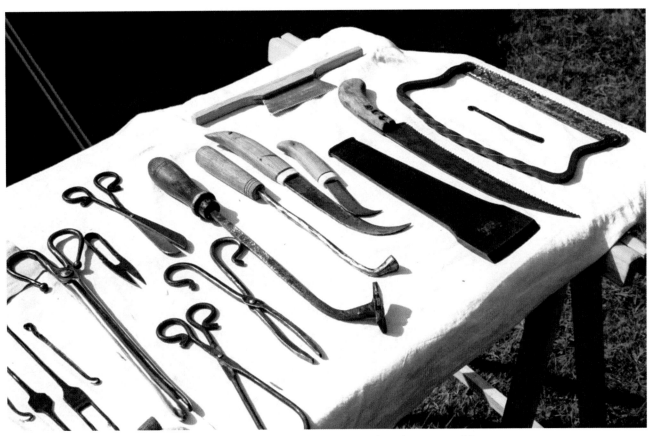

Figure 9.1 Special tools used by medieval surgeons [4].

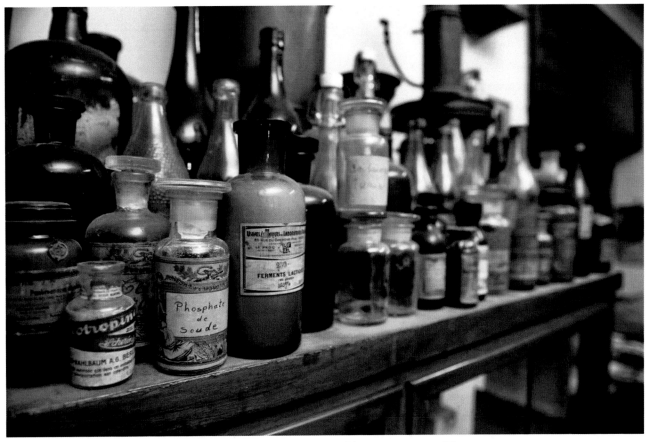

Figure 9.2 Potions produced by wise women [4].

Traditional Arabic and Islamic medicine (TAIM) was developed in medieval times and practiced in various Arabic countries today. It contains ancient healing wisdom and guidelines for healthy living. Past down from generation to generation, the medical herbs, seeds, roots, and oils have been utilized to treat a wide range of illnesses and diseases. Understanding TAIM will enhance the ability of traditional healer to provide culturally sensitive care to Arab and Muslim patients.

This chapter provides an introduction to the traditional medicine commonly used in Arab or Islamic communities. It begins by providing a brief history of TAIM. It discusses what TAIM is all about. It covers Arabic and Islamic herbal medicines. It addresses how Arabic or Islamic medicine is practiced in Arab nations and Islamic communities. It presents some diseases that have been treated by TAIM. It highlights some benefits and challenges of TAIM. The last section concludes with comments.

9.2 BRIEF HISTORY OF ARABIC MEDICINE

Traditional Arabic and Islamic medicine (TAIM) represents the medical tradition that thrived during the Golden Age of Islam. It is a holistic system of medicine which started hundreds of years ago and were used until recently throughout Europe. It refers to medicine developed in the medieval Islamic civilization and mostly written in Arabic, the lingua franca of the Islamic civilization.

Ancient Egypt was a civilization that lasted from 3300 to 525 B.C.E. This is probably where the concept of health started. The ancient Egyptians thought that gods, demons, and spirits played a key role in causing diseases. The Golden Age of Islamic medicine (800 to 1300 CE) is a notable period in medical history.

The Arabian conquests during and after the 7th century led to a spread of Islam and brought back medical skills and remedies, based on the teachings of the Quran on health.

People generally believed that Allah (God) would provide treatment for every illness. By 900 AD, Islamic medicine had become a science in its own right. As people became more interested in health, Islamic doctors strived to find healing procedures that looked at the natural causes and potential treatments or cures. The advent of Islam gave rise to impressive discoveries in many fields, especially medicine. Islamic scholars developed new techniques in medicine, dissection, surgery, and pharmacology. They founded the first hospitals, introduced physician training, and wrote encyclopedias of medical knowledge [5].

Islamic scholars and doctors were building on the work of the medical records of Greeks and Romans and making discoveries in medicine. The Greek figures were known in the Arabic-speaking world and provided the early foundations of the medical art in the Islamic world. The Islamic physicians translated many texts from Greek, Persian, Syriac, Indian, Hebrew, and other languages to Arabic, though Arabic became the lingua franca and Islam the dominant faith. The Arabs became renowned for the practice of medicine. The medieval Islamic world produced some of the greatest medical thinkers in history. Al-Razi and Ibn Sina were two Muslim philosophers of the Islamic golden age who changed the concept of medicine for centuries. Al-Razi studied and analyzed ancient Greek medical collections, discovered the cause of smallpox, and wrote the first book on paediatrics. Ibn-Sina (Avicenna), "father of early modern medicine," became the representative of Islamic medicine mainly through the influence of his famous work, *The Canon of Medicine*. Prophetic medicine was developed during the time of Prophet Muhammad, while Islamic medicine is a continuation of endeavors reaching its peak during the Islamic civilization era, the Islamic Golden Age, spanning the 8th to the 15th Centuries [6,7].

Modern medicine started to emerge after the Industrial Revolution in the 18th century. At this time, there was rapid growth in economic activity in Western Europe and the Americas. The history of Western medicine owes much to its encounters with the medieval Muslim world,

9.3 CONCEPT OF ARABIC TRADITIONAL MEDICINE

The Arabic traditional medicine (also known as Islamic traditional medicine, traditional Arabic and Islamic medicine, or Hilla) is a holistic system of medicine which dates back to 14 centuries ago. It refers to medicine developed in the medieval Islamic civilization and mostly written in Arabic, the lingua franca of the Islamic civilization. Hotness, coldness, moistness, and dryness are four temperaments that naturally occur in every existing substance including living creatures [8].

The traditional Arabic and Islamic medicine (TAIM) is a system of healing practiced since antiquity in the Arab world (Saudi Arabia, Iran, Iraq, Qatar, Egypt, Syria, Pakistan, United Arab Emirates (UAE), etc.). It is the culmination of Graeco-Roman, Chinese, Persian, and Ayurvedic practices. It consists of medicinal herbs, dietary practices, mind-body practices, spiritual healing, and applied therapy. The development of TAIM started with the Prophet. A unified TAIM conceptual model is shown in Figure 9.3.

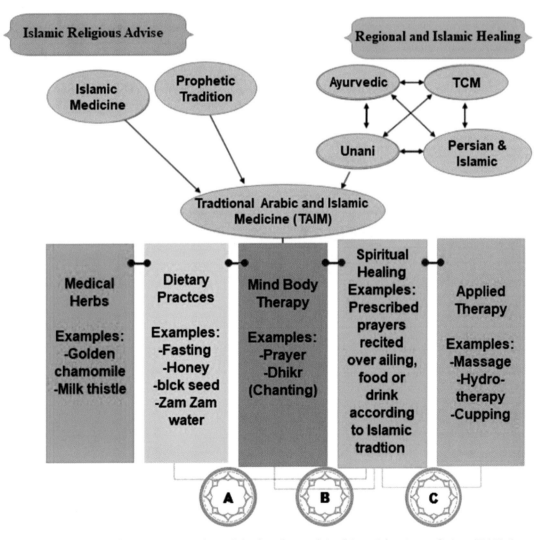

Figure 9.3 A unifying conceptual model of traditional Arabic & Islamic medicine (TAIM).

Medicine of the Prophet is based on the Quran and other Islamic texts and traditional herbal remedies. It is not based on medical experiments but rather on inspiration and accumulated medical knowledge from ancient culture and tradition. According to a Hadith, the stomach is the core of the body and origin of many diseases: "The stomach is the central basin of the body, and the veins are connected to it. When the stomach is healthy, it passes on its condition to veins, and in turn the veins will circulate the same and when the stomach is putrescence. Mohammad's approach to herbal medicine is very much rooted in the humoral concepts. The distinguishing feature of herbal medicine as practiced for purging and adjusting the Four Humors – Blood, Phlegm, Yellow Bile, and Black Bile. The theory held that four different bodily fluids (or humors) influenced human health. Medical establishments believed that levels of these humors would fluctuate in the body, depending on what people ate, drank, inhaled, and what they had been doing. The theory lasted for 2,000 years, until scientists discredited it.

The Muslims put a premium on cleanliness and dietary regime. The ritual cleansing of the body precedes each of the five daily prayers. Disease was regarded as divine punishment for the sins of man. Islam emphasizes on equilibrium among man, his soul, and the universe. All aspects of Islamic thought must conform to Muslim worldview as indicated in the Quran. Knowledge is legitimate so long as it remains within the framework of the worldview. Islamic medicine is closely bound up with the principles of the faith.

From an Islamic perspective, health is considered as the state of physical, psychological, social, and spiritual wellbeing. Health is regarded as one of the greatest blessings of God on humankind. A Muslim patient perceives illness as a trial from God. A disease is viewed as divine punishment for the sins of man. Muslim healers rely on both physical and spiritual means to cure disease and promote wellness. Caring for Muslim patients involves an awareness of the Islamic faith and Islamic beliefs. Muslim patients should be cared for by a nurse of the same gender since touching (or shaking hands) is prohibited between members of the opposite sex, except they are family members [10]. Both the healers and patients generally believe that Allah (God) would provide treatment for every illness. God forbids us to do harm to others and imposes on physicians the oath not to compose harmful remedies. The healers often use verses in the Quran to go along with their treatments. An ancient Muslim healer is shown in Figure 9. 4 [11]. Healing may require dietary practices and prayer. In addition to the obligatory fast of Ramadan, there are various optional fasts for maintaining physical health. Fasting also carries immense spiritual rewards as the desired effects occur in the realm of the soul and its evolution. Water from a well located in Mecca, the holiest place in Islam, can also be used for healing [12].

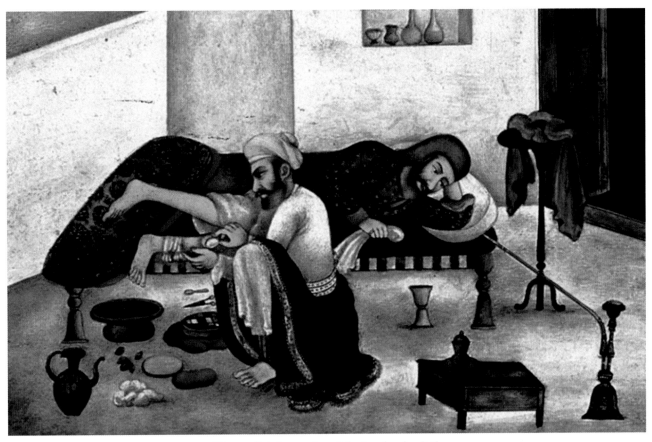

Figure 9.4 An ancient Muslim healer [11].

The Persian physician, Ibn Sina, wrote *The Canon of Medicine*. He explains considerations for testing new medicines, known as the Avicenna's rules:[13]:

1. The drug must be pure and not contain anything that would reduce its quality.
2. The investigator must test the drug on one simple disease, not a condition that could have various complications.
3. They should test the medication on at least two distinct diseases, because sometimes a drug might treat one disease effectively and another one by accident.
4. A drug's quality must match the severity of the disease. For example, if the "heat" of a drug is less than the "coldness" of a disease, it will not work.
5. The researcher must time the process carefully, so that the action of the drug is not confused with other confounding factors, such as the natural healing process.
6. The drug's effect must be consistent with several trials showing the same results. In this way, the investigator can rule out any accidental effects.
7. Investigators must test the drug on humans, not animals, as it may not work in the same way for both.

9.4 ARABIC HERBS

Arab and Muslim scholars introduced hundreds of natural products, especially medicinal plants. Many plants and animal products are mentioned in the Holy Quran. Muslims have always sought the Quran as a healing source in times of illness. Herbal medicines are very common in the Arab world. They play a significant role in disease management in Arabic nations. Herbs were produced to resolve each imbalance humor. Without access to medical doctors, people have relied on herbs, amulets, and invocations. There are roughly 250 plant species currently used in traditional Arabic medicine for treating various diseases. Figure 9.5 shows some Arab herds in display [14]. Common Arab herds include [15,16]:

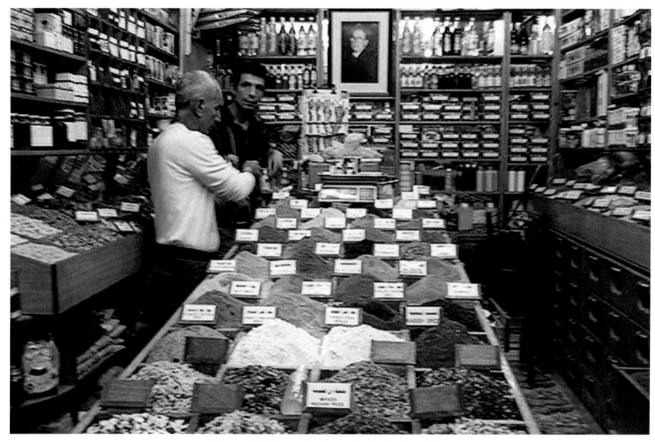

Figure 9.5 Some Arab herds in display [14].

- *Saffron* (Crocus sativus L.): This is a spece belonging to the Iridaceae family and is widely used as an herbal medicine, spice, food coloring, and a flavoring agent since ancient times. This plant has also been used for the treatment of impotence and female genito-urinary system disorders.
- *Olive Oil:* This is renowned for its healthy fatty acids, skin-softening, and heart-protective qualities. The leaf extracts has anti-inflammatory, anti-bacterial and anti-fungal properties, making it a well-rounded and powerful supplement.
- *Anise Oil:* This helps with cough and flu cases and improves digestion, alleviates cramps, and reduces nausea. If taken in high doses, anise oil can be used as an antiseptic and for the treatment of asthma and bronchitis.
- *Pomegranate:* This has been used for its astringent effects and to treat numerous ailments including sore throat, inflammation, digestive and bladder issues. Pomegranate juice selectively inhibits the growth of breast, colon, and lung cancer cells.
- *Thyme:* This is a very popular herb used in food, wounds, diarrhea, stomach ache, arthritis, sore throats, and for treatment for respiratory, inflammatory, and digestive conditions. It is also used as

a treatment for respiratory, inflammatory, and digestive conditions. It smells wonderfully fragrant in cooking. A tea made from the leaves is also a popular remedy against cough, cold, and flu.

- *Black Cumin:* The black cumin seed is attributed to have amazing health benefits. The Prophet Muhammad once said that black cumin is "the remedy for all diseases except death." Black cumin seeds have high amount of health benefits. They are shown in Figure 9.6 [17].

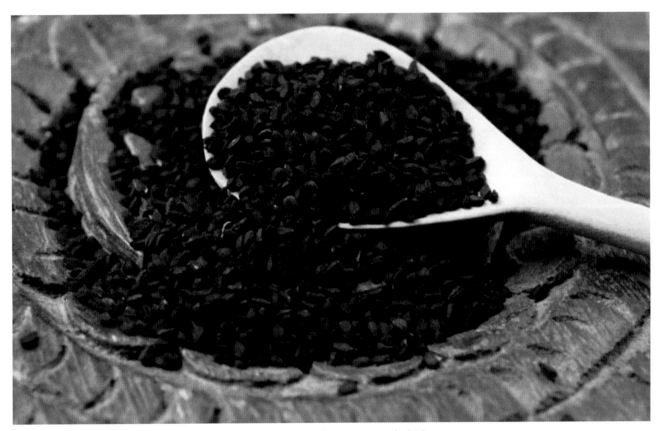

Figure 9.6 Black cumim seeds [17].

- *Aloe Vera:* This is used in ancient Egyptian times to heal burns and skin diseases. Other conditions and treatments include pain, vomiting, asthma, burns, skin disease, and epilepsy.
- *Gum Arabic:* It has been used in herbal medicine since ancient times. It fights colds and coughs, helps treat sore throats, gonorrhea patients, and leprosy. It promotes digestive health and helps overcome digestive problems.
- *Zallouh:* This plant has been used since ancient times as a mild tonic remedy. It may have a role in increasing sexual energy and improving potency in sexual dysfunction.
- *Onion* (Allium cepa): This is another plant mentioned in the verses and hadiths of Islam religion. The plant has several therapeutic properties. An Arabic scholar has said, "Eat onion because there are three benefits for the onion: it makes your mouth fragrant, tightens the gum, and increases the amount of semen and sexual intercourse."
- *Honey:* This is recommended in the Quran for internal use and is widely used in folk traditions. It has been used as a wound dressing. It is the best treatment for the gums and many diseases. Muslim patients with diabetes may use honey as a traditional remedy.
- *Cannabis and Opium:* Doctors prescribed these, but only for therapeutic purposes, as they realized that they were powerful drugs.

- *Turmeric:* This contains the chemical curcumin that decreases inflammation in the body. The spice also functions as a very potent antioxidant.
- *St John's Wort:* This is a significant element of Arab herbal medicine heritage that was used by practitioners in Palestine, the usage of this plant in the region has become almost extinct.

9.5 ARABIC MEDICINE IN MUSLIM NATIONS

Arabic or Islamic medicine is practiced in Arab nations and communities in South East Asia, the Indian subcontinent, Central Asian countries, the Middle East, the Horn of Africa, and North and West African. Research and development of the traditional medicinal herbs has been conducted in many Arab nations such as Saudi Arabia, Iran, Iraq, Qatar, Egypt, Pakistan, United Arab Emirates (UAE), Syria, Morocco, Indonesia, Palestine, Yemen, and others. Muslims from different parts of the world will have varying cultures even though they share the same religious beliefs. There is a great diversity of cultural, ethnic, and linguistic groups within Muslim countries, each of which has its own cultural characteristics and world view of health and illness. Although there are Western-oriented Muslims who may or may not adhere strictly to the practices of Islam, Islamic practices dominate every aspect of most Muslims. We consider how the following nations practice TAIM.

- *Saudi Arabia:* The Kingdom of Saudi Arabia has made a tremendous progress in its healthcare system in the past few decades. This Muslim country is witnessing a healthcare transformation as a part of the Saudi 2030 vision and facing some challenges. Healthcare challenges in Saudi Arabia include increased burden of noncommunicable diseases, maintaining quality healthcare services, avoiding a supply gap, back and neck pain, depressive disorders, migraine, diabetes, cancer, and anxiety disorders. The TAIM is being used by a substantial proportion of Saudis but like a shadow healthcare system. This phenomenon of using two healthcare systems reflects a need for an integrative healthcare system. The objective of integrative medicine is to include the best practices of both conventional and complementary therapy, uniting these practices into an integrative approach. The search for an alternative healing system to respond to the unmet need in modern medicine is an additional motivation [18].
- *Qatar:* Within the past two decades, Qatar has been transformed from a relatively unknown Gulf State to a prominent player on the world stage. In the process, Qatar has exploited its significant oil and gas reserves. Qatar is planning to have the world's first center for Traditional Arabic Islamic Medicine (TAIM), at the Zulal Wellness Resort, opening in 2022. As the use of traditional medicine continues to gain momentum around the world, Zulal Wellness Resort is set to bring TAIM to the forefront of the wellness industry in Qatar. The aim is for new venture to attract international visitors seeking health and wellness [19,20].
- *United Arab Emirates* (UAE): In this Arab nation, the use of herbal medicine among the citizens has become prevalent. Herbal remedy is freely available to all residents through from retail outlets. A large number of unregistered herbal products is dispensed from wide range of outlets. A notable practice in UAE is the increased prevalence for the self medication, along with concomitant use of herbal and conventional medicines [21].
- *Northern Nigeria:* This part of Nigeria is inhabited predominantly by Hausas and Fulanis. The Hausa traditional practitioner/malam has the reputation of being an effective and intelligent

healer. His understanding of herbs and the healing properties of the Quran is reputedly superb. The medicine is based on the Quran. There are now many Islamized African societies in which there are three and not two medical systems operating side by side: a traditional pre-Islamic, an Islamic, and a Western system. For decades, medicinal plants and herbal practices have been used to treat infectious and other non-infectious diseases in Nigeria [22,23].

9.6 APPLICATIONS OF ARABIC TRADITIONAL MEDICINE

Arabic traditional medicine has become a part of modern life in the Middle East, and it is acquiring worldwide respect. TAIM therapies have shown remarkable success in healing acute as well as chronic diseases and have been utilized by people in most countries of the Mediterranean who have faith in spiritual healers. Arab medical herbalists treat everything from infertility to impotence to heart problems with leaves and other medical products. The following examples are diseases that TAIM can cure:

- *Cancer:* Cancer is a leading cause of death worldwide. The incidence of cancer is increasing in both developed countries and developing nations. Cancer is due to abnormalities in the DNA of the affected cells leading to an extra mass of tissue called a tumor. There are several Islamic and Arabic herbs used for treating cancer. Each plant has been investigated for its anticancer potential [24]. The use of traditional medicine is very common worldwide among people with cancer. The medicine is applied at different stages of the diagnosis and treatment.
- *COVID-19:* There have been several declarations on the use of herbal-based traditional medicine for the prevention or definitive diagnosis of coronavirus disease 2019 (COVID-19). Many of the claims are difficult to verify because of the lack of documented evidence showing that these remedies prevent suffering from COVID-19. As the pandemic continues to spread, there are increasing messages promoting the use of herbal-based traditional medicines for COVID-19. Currently, no herbal remedy has been validated for use to prevent or treat COVID19 [25].
- *Dehydration:* This is a serious problem in the hot desert. To avoid heat exhaustion and heat stroke, one should stay in shade as much as possible. Heat exhaustion is characterized by severe fatigue, headaches, confusion, nausea, weak pulse, cold clammy skin, and giddiness. Heat stroke is a very dangerous and potentially fatal condition characterized by a high body temperature and no sweating. People with heat stroke need immediate hospitalization; and should be cooled with wet towels until then. A local means of treating dehydration is squeezing some lemon or add a tablespoon of apple cider vinegar to your glass of water and drink it slowly, compensating for daily dehydration.
- *Fasting:* This is a therapy on its own. When done properly, fasting has a significant number of benefits. Fasting can lead to weight loss, aid digestive system, activate brain function, and improve focus and concentration. Fasting also has a special place in the framework of the holistic approach. Fasting is one the fundamental tenants of Islam and the primary fast is called Ramadan, the Muslim month of fasting. Ramadan is a unique time, combining therapeutical effect on human body and mind. Ramadan embodies the philosophy of holistic wellness, giving an equal importance to body, mind, and spirit [26]. This fast requires restraining the eyes from immoral sight and the tongue from obscenity.

- *Infertility:* This has been a disease that has been problematic to both men and women for a long time. Infertility is regarded as an illness, one that could be cured if the proper steps are taken. The treatment for infertility by Arab medical experts often depends on the type of conception theory they follow. The prevention and treatment of male infertility are based on the medicinal plants. Increasing men's health and sexual power can reduce the number of divorces caused by women's dissatisfaction. Treatments used by followers of this method often include treating infertile women with substances that are similar to fertilizer. One example of such a treatment is the insertion of fig juice into the womb [27].

- *Overweight:* This is a major challenge worldwide, especially in the Western world. It often leads to serious clinical complications such as type 2 diabetes mellitus and heart diseases. Effective management of overweight seems to be of utmost importance. Available pharmacological therapy of obesity is limited to few with side effects. A mixture of extract of four plants used in traditional Arabic and Islamic medicine has been prepared and assessed for its safety and efficacy in weight loss. This plant combination has no anti-overweight effects [28].

Other health issues that have been treated by Arabic medicine include miscarriage, contraception, menstrual pain, smallpox, leprosy, and depression.

9.7 BENEFITS

TAIM refers to healing practices and philosophy incorporating herbal medicines, spiritual therapies, dietary practices, and mind-body techniques. The Arab world has known how to use natural remedies for millennia. Past down from generation to generation, these herbs, seeds, roots and oils have been used to cure countless people before modern medicine was invented. Herbal treatments are the most commonly utilized form of traditional medicine. They are lucrative in the international market. Herbal remedies carry an emotional message of cultural empowerment. Arabic medicine has made a major contribution to the development of pharmacy. Many of the herbs have been tested in clinical studies within the Arab communities.

Other benefits include:

- *Easy Access to Healthcare:* Traditional medicine provides a platform for ensuring that all people have access to care. TAIM therapies have shown remarkable success in treating chronic diseases and is the first choice for many in dealing with ailments such as infertility, epilepsy, psychosomatic troubles, and depression.

- *Economic Benefit:* Arabic traditional medicines are lucrative in the international market. A successful medicine business is an invaluable way of raising the profile and value of locally grown herbs. This will also aid farmers, herbal experts, and all those involved in Arabic medicine.

- *Holistic Treatment:* TAIM encompasses a holistic approach to wellness based on the traditional Arabic principles, which have influenced and inspired the development of modern medicine. Holistic wellness acknowledges the importance of temporary food deprivation to reset the mind. Individualized, holistic care can only be achieved by understanding culture, beliefs, and traditions.

- *Ethics:* This is important in Islamic medicine. It is important not only for the physician to be an expert in his field, but he must also to be a role model. Traditional medical ethics can be divided into three concepts: the physician's responsibility to patients and to self, and also the patients' responsibility to physicians. Muslim physicians have put much emphasis on ethical principles in their practice. For thousands of years, ethics are required as an essential requirement in the making of a physician.

9.8 CHALLENGES

When traditional physicians do not know how to cure a disease, they often turn to superstitious rites and magic. Since Arabic is the lingua franca of the Islamic world, some traditional medicines used to be in Arabic and that prevented their global adoption. There is increasing concern about the safety of medicinal plants. Many medicinal herbs are therapeutic at one dose and toxic at another. The exact dose of traditional medicine is often variable or unknown. Several cases of contamination and poisons were detected in vegetables and plant in Arab world such as Morocco, Egypt, Iraq, Saudi Arabia, Sudan, Syria, Jordan, UAE, Pakistan, and Yemen in the recent years [29].

Other challenges include [8]:

- *Danger of Extinction:* A serious problem is that many herbs used in Arabic traditional medicine are now rare. Medicinal herbs are great resources for various pharmaceutical compounds and should be protected from natural destruction and disappearance. This may cause the danger of indigenous Arab medicinal practices and knowledge disappearing altogether. Many plant herbs used in traditional medicine are now rare or endangered species. Our heritage of plant herbs that flourished a few centuries ago is now in rapid decline. Factors endangering plant herbs include habitat loss, habitat degradation, overharvesting, detrimental climatic, and environmental changes.

- *Transmitting Knowledge:* The occupation of traditional healer is a family matter and passed on by inheritance. The process of transmitting traditional medical knowledge from one generation is complex. Most practitioners have very limited knowledge in the identification of species and procedures for preparing medicinal remedies. Younger practitioners are less experienced than their older counterparts, indicating that traditional knowledge is being partially lost with new generations. The level of education of practitioners is in decline, indicating that the traditional medical practice may disappear in some regions of the Middle East.

- *Decline in Herbal Knowledge:* There has been a decline in the great knowledge and use of herbs in the Arab world, mostly as a result of the increased availability of modern medicine. Due to urbanization changes in lifestyles in the Middle East, the knowledge of the uses of Medicinal plants for healing purposes has been lost.

- *Toxicity:* There are concerns regarding toxicity and adverse effects of traditional remedies. Many medicinal herbs therapeutic at one dose and toxic at another. Toxicity related to traditional medicines is becoming more widely recognized worldwide. Most reports concerning the toxic effects of herbal medicines are associated with hepatotoxicity.

- *Regulations:* There are no governmental regulations on the manufacture, concentration, or labeling claims of herbal medicines. Islamic religious regulations on hygiene have led to the creation of special control services. In the US, most herbal products are considered dietary supplements and are not required to meet the stringent standards.

These challenges are displayed in Figure 9.7.

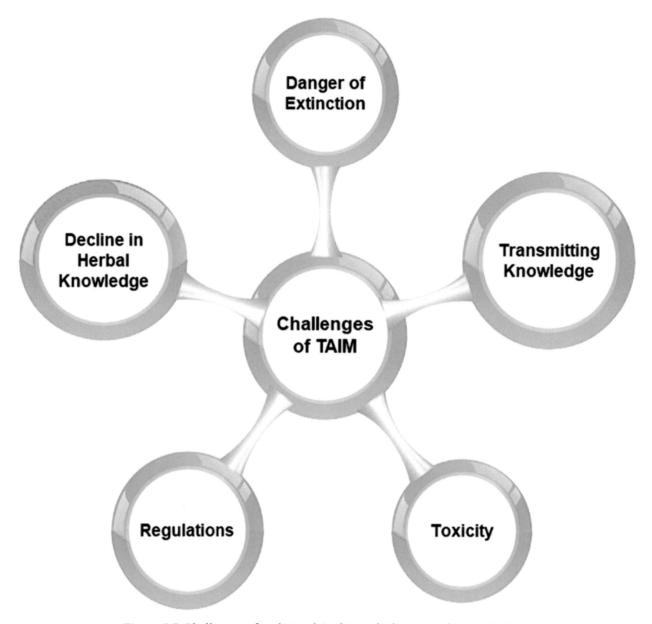

Figure 9.7 Challenges of traditional Arabic and Islamic medicine (TAIM).

9.9 GLOBALIZATION OF ARABIC MEDICINE

In the last decades, traditional medicine has attracted the interest of the global researchers. As the present, over 80% of the world population depends on traditional medicines. As a result, attention to traditional, complementary applications of medicine is on the rise. For decades, World Health Organization (WHO) has been trying to revive traditional medical practices globally. Traditional medicine has become either the mainstay of healthcare delivery or serves as a complement. The WHO, China, India, Nigeria, and the US have invested considerably in traditional herbal medicines research, a significant step towards global health.

Although there are currently no Arab traditional medicine training programs in any Arab country, global use of Arabic traditional medicine has continued to gain momentum. As a global religion, Islam along with Islamic medicine is practiced within various cultural milieus. Islamic medicine and beauty products have become a big business worldwide. The Arabic or Islamic traditional medicine is used in a lot of nations, especially Muslin nations. Nations throughout the Middle East including Egypt, Jordan, and the Arabian Gulf have started incorporating TAIM along with conventional medicine [9].

9.10 CONCLUSION

Arabic-speaking world provided the early foundations of the medical art in the Islamic world. Traditional Arabic Islamic Medicine (TAIM) evolved from Graeco-Roman, Chinese, Persian, and Ayurvedic medical practices. It refers to the science of medicine developed in the Islamic Golden Age and written in Arabic. It is the system of healing practiced since antiquity in the Arab world with the influence of Islam. TAIM incorporates herbal medicines, spiritual therapies, dietary practices, and manual techniques.

In recent times, traditional medicine has become the interest of the global researchers. There is a growing body of knowledge on the role of various dietary plants in reducing disease. The Arab world has known how to use natural remedies for centuries. The knowledge of herbal remedies in Arabic (Islamic) medicine is vast.

The traditional medicine is increasingly being used in nations where allopathic medicine is predominant in the healthcare system. Arabic-speaking world provided the early foundations of the medical art in the Islamic world. More information about Persian traditional medicine can be found in the books in [30-43] and related journals:

- *Journal of Integrative Medicine*
- *Journal of Medicinal Plants Research*
- *Current Traditional Medicine*
- *Traditional Medicine Research*
- *Journal of Traditional and Complementary Medicine*
- *Journal of Complementary Medicine & Alternative Healthcare*
- *International Journal on Complementary and Alternative Medicine*
- *Traditional and Integrative Medicine*
- *Evidence-Based Complementary and Alternative Medicine*

REFERENCES

[1]   B. Saad and O. Said, "Natural drugs in Greco-Arabic and Islamic medicine," November 2020, https://muslimheritage.com/natural-drugs-in-greco-arabic-and-islamic-medicine/

[2]   M. N. O. Sadiku, U. C. Chukwu, A. Ajayi-Majebi, S. M. Musa, "Traditional Arabic and Islamic medicine: An overview," *International Journal of Trend in Scientific Research and Development*, vol. 6, no. 1, November- December 2021, pp.1014–1019.

[3]   H. Edriss et al., "Islamic medicine in the middle ages," *The American Journal of the Medical Sciences*, vol. 354, no. 3, September 2017, pp. 223-229.

[4]   "What was medieval and renaissance medicine?" https://www.medicalnewstoday.com/articles/323533#middle-ages

[5] P. Johnstone, "Tradition in Arabic medicine," *Palestine Exploration Quarterly*, vol. 107, no. 1, 1975, pp. 23-37.

[6] I. R. Ibrahim et al., "The history of traditional medicine in the Arab region," *International Journal on Complementary and Alternative Medicine*, vol. 4, no. 2, December 2017.

[7] "6 Important Islamic achievements in medieval medicine," December 2021, https://www.historyonthenet.com/6-important-islamic-achievements-in-medieval-medicine

[8] B. Javadi, A. Sahebkar, and S. A. Emami, "A survey on saffron in major Islamic traditional medicine books," *Iran Journal of Basic Medical Science,* vol. 16, no. 1, January 2013, pp. 1-11.

[10] G. H. Rassool, "Cultural competence in nursing Muslim patients," *Nursing Times,* vol. 111, no. 14 March 2015, pp. 12-15.

[11] "Revival of the natural sciences: Tibb in the 21st Century," October 2015, https://www.bahath.co/revival-of-the-natural-sciences/tibb-in-the-21st-century

[12] S. Al-Rawi and M. D. Fetters, "Traditional Arabic & Islamic medicine: A conceptual model for clinicians and researchers," *Global Journal of Health Science,* vol. 4, no. 3, May 2012, pp.164–169.

[13] "Why was medieval Islamic medicine important?" https://www.medicalnewstoday.com/articles/323612

[14] D. Osborn, "My healing journey in the Holy Land, " June 2010, http://www.greekmedicine.net/blog/herbs/my-healing-journey-in-the-holy-land.html

[15] "The six: Traditional natural remedies from the Middle East," October 2018, https://www.arabnews.com/node/1387891/food-health

[16] "Healing herbs: Seven ancient plant remedies from the Arab world," November 2021, https://www.middleeasteye.net/discover/home-remedies-cold-seven-traditional-arab-world

[17] "Traditional natural remedies from the Middle East," https://www.abouther.com/node/14181/lifestyle/health-nutrition/traditional-natural-remedies-middle-east

[18] M. K. Khalil et al., "The future of integrative health and medicine in Saudi Arabia," *Integrative Medicine Research,* vol. 7, no. 4, December 2018, pp. 316-321.

[19] "Rediscovering traditional Arabic and Islamic medicine at Zulal Wellness Resort," November 2021, https://thepeninsulaqatar.com/article/28/09/2020/Rediscovering-traditional-medicine-at-Zulal-Wellness-Resort

[20] "Qatar's traditional Arabic Islamic medicine plan," April 2021, https://www.laingbuissonnews.com/imtj/news-imtj/qatars-traditional-arabic-islamic-medicine-plan/

[21] S. A. Fahmy, S. Abdu, and M. Abuelkhair, "Pharmacists' attitude, perceptions and knowledge towards the use of herbal products in Abu Dhabi, United Arab Emirates," *Pharmacy Practice (Internet),* vol. 8, no. 2, April-June, 2010, pp. 109-115.

[22] I. H. Abdalla, "Islamic medicine and its influence on traditional Hausa practitioners in northern Nigeria," *Doctoral Dissertation,* University of Wisconsin-Madison, August 1981.

[23] I. B. Abubakar et al., "Traditional medicinal plants used for treating emerging and re-emerging viral diseases in northern Nigeria," *European Journal of Integrative Medicine,* vol. 49, 2022.

[24] H. Zaid et al., "Cancer treatment by Greco-Arab and Islamic herbal medicine," *The Open Nutraceuticals Journal,* vol. 3, 2010, pp. 203-212.

[25] "Statement on herbal remedies and medicines for prevention and treatment of COVID-19," https://africacdc.org/download/statement-on-herbal-remedies-and-medicines-for-prevention-and-treatment-of-covid-19-2/

[26] "Zulal wellness resort provides advice on maintaining a balanced wellness routine for a healthy and peaceful month of Ramadan," April 2021, https://www.dunesmagazine.com/post/zulal-wellness-resort-shares-traditional-arabic-islamic-medicine-inspired-wellness-tips-this-ramadan

[27] "Medicine in the medieval Islamic world," *Wikipedia,* the free encyclopedia https://en.wikipedia.org/wiki/Medicine_in_the_medieval_Islamic_world

[28] O. Said et al., "Weight loss in animals and humans treated with 'weighlevel', a combination of four medicinal plants used in traditional Arabic and Islamic medicine," *Evidence-Based Complementary and Alternative Medicine,* 2011.

[29] B. Saad et al., "Safety of traditional Arab herbal medicine," *Evidence-Based Complementary and Alternative Medicine,* vol. 3, no. 4, December 2006, pp. 433-439.

[30] G. Bos, *Maimonides, on the Regimen of Health: A New Parallel Arabic-English Translation (Medical Works of Moses Maimonides).* Brill, 2019.

[31] B. Saad and O. Said, *Greco-Arab and Islamic Herbal Medicine: Traditional System, Ethics, Safety, Efficacy, and Regulatory Issues.* John Wiley & Sons, 2011.

[32] P. E. Pormann and E. Savage-Smith, *Medieval Islamic Medicine.* Edinburgh University Press, 2007.

[33] S. A. Ghazanfar, *Handbook of Arabian Medicinal Plants.* Boca Raton, FL: CRC Press, 1994.

[34] Y. A. Ahmad, *Islamic Medicine - The Key to a Better Life.* Darul Salaam, 2009.

[35] The Editorial Team, *Botany, Herbals and Healing In Islamic Science and Medicine.* Independently Published, 2009.

[36] H. A. Qadeer, *Unani: The Science of Graeco-Arabic Medicine.* Lustre Press - Roli Books, 1998.

[37] M. S. Khan, *Islamic Medicine.* Routledge, 2013.

[38] M. Ullman, *Islamic Medicine.* Edinburgh University Press, 1978.

[39] Y. A. Ahmad and N. Al-Khattab (eds.), *The Islamic Guideline on Medicine.* Dar-us-Salam Publications, 2010.

[40] J. A. Morrow, *Encyclopedia of Islamic Herbal Medicine.* McFarland & Company, 2011.

[41] I. Q. Al-Jawziyya, *Medicine of the Prophet.* Islamic Texts Society, 1998.

[42] S. Alavi, *Islam and Healing: Loss and Recovery of an Indo-Muslim Medical Tradition, 1600-1900.* Permanent Black, 2007.

[43] Z. Amar and E. Lev, *Arabian Drugs in Early Medieval Mediterranean Medicine (Edinburgh Studies in Classical Islamic History and Culture).* Edinburgh University Press, 2016.

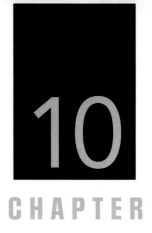

CHAPTER

Mexician Traditonal Medicine

"Nature itself is the best physicians." - Hippocrates

10.1 INTRODUCTION

Since ancient times, humanity has used herbal plants to cure disease in all cultures. Humans have used plants to satisfy many of their needs as food and also to obtain relief from illness and disease. It is well known that modern medicine is desperately short of new treatments. It takes years for a new drug to be developed, go through rigorous laboratory tests, get approved, and become commercialized. Today, many scientists have started to search indigenous sources for new drugs.

The World Health Organization (WHO) has called for the protection of traditional knowledge, the integration of alternative medicine in national health systems, and the certification of those who practice traditional healing. Traditional medicine is a set of beliefs, knowledge, and practices, from popular culture, used to solve health problems. Traditional medicine is practiced in rural communities in Mexico where modern healthcare is limited or difficult to access [1] The traditional medical services improve the quality of life of the patients through both physical and emotional care. The efficacy of the herbal medicines that Mexicans bring from Mexico to the United States is well documented. In terms of rich ancestral traditional medicinal knowledge, Mexico is recognized as the second most important nation in the world, just after China.

People of Latin-American descent, now more commonly called Latinos, are among the fastest growing ethnic groups of the US population. Latinos constitute almost 13% of the US population. Although Mexican-Americans were initially living in southwestern states, they now live throughout the entire nation. Like other immigrant groups, the Mexicans cherish their family recipes and embrace their culture through food, fiestas, and family life [2]. The population of Mexico is roughly 130 millions. As typically shown in Figure 10.1, festivals and fiestas are extremely important in Mexico and celebrated even in the villages [3]. The Mexican culture is rich with traditions that are well documented to have existed long before Columbus sailed the ocean blue. The earliest Mexican settlers in Chicago expressed distrust of modern doctors and the medicines they offered.

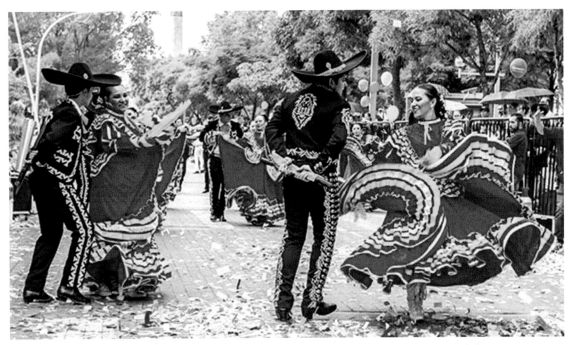

Figure 10.1 Festivals and fiestas are extremely important in Mexico [3].

Traditional medicines are very important in Mexico. The traditional medicine from ancient Mesoamerica by way of Mexico can teach us today about well-being and healing in mind, body, spirit, and emotions. It is one of the many types of alternative or folk medicine practitioners among the Hispanic community. Figure 10.2 shows the map of Mesoamerica [4]. Traditional Mexican healing practices have survived conquest, colonization, and modern medicine because many modalities require little if any equipment. Mexico is regarded for its cultural and biological diversity, which is reflected in the vast traditional knowledge of herbal remedies [5].

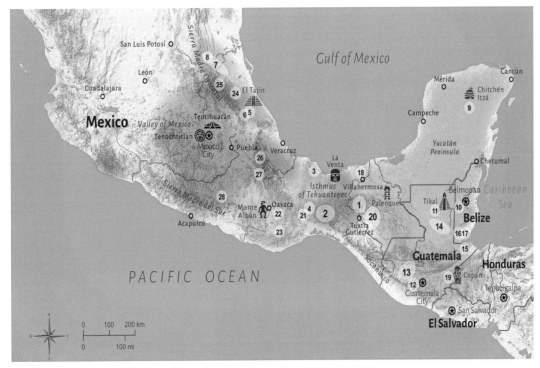

Figure 10.2 Map of Mesoamerica [4].

This chapter provides an introduction on Mexican traditional medicine (MTM). It begins by providing a brief history about MTM. It explains the concept of MTM. It discusses some Mexican herbs. It gives some applications of MTM in treating some diseases. It highlights the benefits and challenges of MTM. It covers globalization of Mexican medicine. The last section concludes with comments.

10.2 BRIEF HISTORY OF MEXICAN MEDICINE

This is by no means a comprehensive history. The Mexican culture is rich with alternative health system which has its origins in ancient Mestizo/Indian folklore. Ancient Mesopotamia, which is the modern-day Middle East, is where the oldest texts about traditional medicine were found and sourced back to about 2100 BCE. Ancient Egyptians also contributed greatly to traditional medicine by about 1700 BCE, when they prescribed medicinal plants for certain ailments. There are significant civilizations of ancient Mexico that were also known for their alternative medicine practices [6].

Mexican traditional medicine (MTM) originates from pre-Columbian Mexican culture. It shares similar characteristics with other Latino traditional healing practices. It has served as the basis for indigenous healing practices for more than 400 years. Prior to the arrival of the Spaniards in 1519, Mexico was the home of the highly sophisticated and spiritually based Aztec civilization, which boasted vast knowledge of healing herbs. In Aztec society, the upper class was composed of priests, nobles, and officers. The lower class was composed of artisans, vendors, soldiers, and farmers. Every aspect of Aztec life was grounded in religious belief and practice. An Aztec physician knew the curative power of plants, trees, roots and rocks, knew the benefits of massage, could reduce fractures, heal wounds, and make incisions. Women were not allowed to practice medicine.

In 1519, when the Spaniards arrived in Mexico, they found that the Aztec civilization was remarkably advanced. A Spanish colonial government was established in Mexico, with the indigenous population converted to Catholicism and the Spanish language, which lasted for a period of over 300 years. The Spanish friars accepted the Aztec medicines with skepticism. The Spanish church saw the Aztec gods and religious practices as evil. As a result, 3,000 medicinal plants were destroyed. Aztec written records (codices) were also destroyed in an attempt to do away with the indigenous culture. In 1552, Martin de la Cruz, Aztec Indian doctor, wrote first book listing 251 herbs. Physicians experimented with hundreds of medical herbs [7,8].

Although some commonly used ingredients have Asian, European, or Middle Eastern roots, they were incorporated into indigenous Mexican healing practices during colonization and continue to be used today. Scholarly investigation made in Mexico in 1994 and 1999 recorded more than a thousand species of medicinal plants with recognized uses.

10.3 CONCEPT OF MEXICAN TRADITIONAL MEDICINE

In order to meet his basic needs, man has always had a close relationship with traditional herbs. Traditional medicine is recognized and promoted by the World Health Organization as an important healthcare resource. Traditional medicine has long been popular in Mexico. With the increase of healthcare costs in the US, many people are seeking alternative means to treat themselves. With traditional medicine, there is no need for an appointment and no need to travel long distances from rural to urban centers. For these reasons, there is a rising movement to restore ancient herbal healing practices.

The traditions and customs of the Mexican people are diverse. They are proud of their native heritage and each region has its own cultural practices and celebrations. There are several indigenous groups within Mexico and have all influenced the Mexican culture in terms of cuisine, medicine, rituals, and language. These indigenous peoples believe that disease exists not only in the people's body but also in their spirit. The Mexican traditional medicine (MTM) approaches tend to be more preventative and lifestyle-oriented than allopathic approaches. Mexicans have a lot of faith in the traditional remedies.

Folk medicine (or curanderismo or medicine of the people) is an alternate system of healthcare that is still widely practiced throughout the US. It is the mixture of traditional healing practices that involve herbal medicine, spirituality, and manual therapies in order to diagnose, treat or prevent illness, and prescribe remedy. Folk remedies are still used to treat illness every day. The healing may consist of rituals, herbal remedies, potions or counter-magic, depending upon the illness being treated. Healing often occurs in a ceremony called a barrida (the "sweeping") where eggs, lemons, and various herbs, along with prayer, are often used.

One of the largest and most widely used systems of folk medicine in the Mexican-American community is called *curanderismo*. This is sometimes known as non-traditional medicine or faith healing. *Curanderismo* is the Spanish term which means "to heal" or "to cure." It describes traditional medicine from ancient Mesoamerica and currently practiced by many communities in Mexico, Central America, and the Amazon. It was influenced by medieval and European witchcraft, early Arabic medicine, and Judeo-Christian religious beliefs.It is a practice that blends Mayan, Aztec, and Spanish Catholic traditions. It is a practice with pre-Hispanic roots that often incorporates prayers to Cathoic saints. *Curanderismo*, traditional folk medicine, can fill a huge void left between modern traditional medicine and the option of receiving no medical treatment. The new health care plan may very well further increase the demand for non-traditional services. Faith healing goes hand in hand with traditional medicine. Most non-traditional practices take place in the patient's home and not in the sterile environment of a doctor's office or a hospital [9].

Mexican traditional healers (or folk healers, or *curanderos*) believe that their healing abilities are a spiritual vocation. The healers understand the connection between good sanitation and good health. *Curanderos* employ many ancient rituals and materials to heal one's body. They use herbs and other plants, incense, and chanting in order to cure illness and travel to spiritual dimensions. Healers of Mexico's indigenous communities want to preserve traditional knowledge and skills on medicinal plants. They intend to pass along herbal healing traditions handed down through the generations. Many healers also offer spiritual counseling services and cleansing rituals. A traditional healer is shown in Figure 10.3 [10].

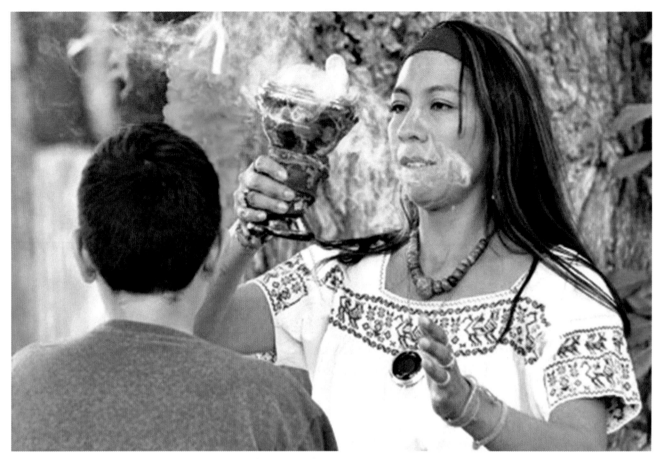

Figure 10.3 A certified traditional healer [10].

10.4 MEXICAN HERBS

Mexico has numerous indigenous herbs that can be used for healing. Studies on herbs from Mexican plants used in traditional medicine have evidenced a great potential for their use as preservatives, antioxidant sources, and functional agents. Many of the herbs are widely available, relatively inexpensive, and effective. They are readily available in marketplaces in Mexico. Herbal teas come in a variety of delicious flavors and they offer health-promoting results. They are therapeutic products and foods made from the leaves, seeds, flowers, and roots of plants, or their extracts. Figure 10.4 shows some Mexican herbs on display [11]. The most widely used are about 50 herbs and there are more than 3,000 species of plants in daily use. Some popular herbs advised for certain conditions are the following [9,12,13]:

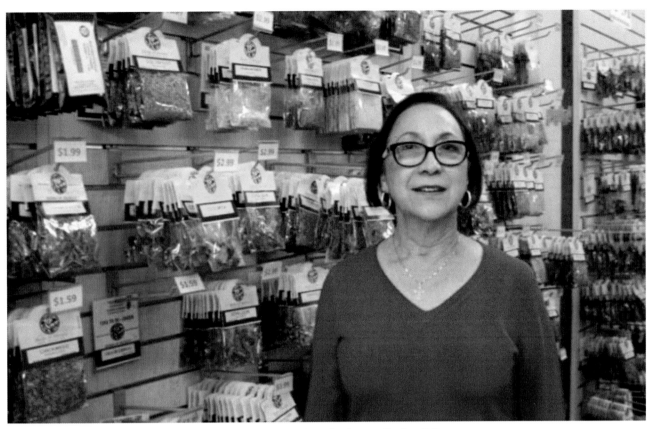

Figure 10.4 Mexican herbs on display [11].

- *Chamomile/manzanilla* is one of the most common natural aids for anxiety, mild depression, and high blood pressure. Chamomile tea has soothing, calming, and relaxing properties. It is a great tea to drink after dinner, before bedtime.
- *Hierbabuena* (mint tea) relieves digestive symptoms, such as gas, bloating, and indigestion.
- *Limes/limones* is used as a diuretic, for sore throats, coughs, and colds. Mexicans put limes on practically everything.
- *Ruda* can help relieve headache or stomach cramps. It also may be used to help with fainting spells and is also used to get rid of piojos (head lice).
- *Zarzamora* is for control of diarrhea and is said to help with general health of the gums.
- *Damiana* helps digestion as well as being an aphrodisiac.
- *Sábila* is a plant with milky, sticky substance that, when applied directly to the affected area, can do wonders for burns. It is said to aid in digestion and can combat infection.
- *Calendula* is a centuries-old antifungal, antiseptic, wound-healing ally.
- *Cilandro* boasts a unique flavor and is a powerful digestive aid that is capable of removing heavy metals and other toxic agents from the body. The seeds are a prime ingredient in Indian curries. Cilandro is shown in Figure 10.5 [12].

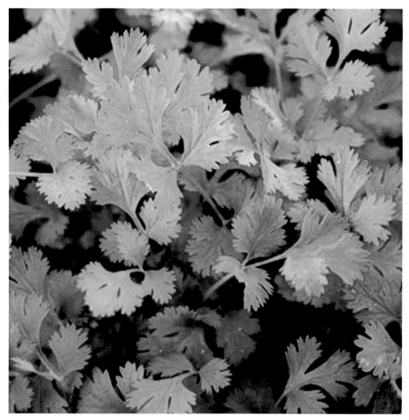

Figure 10.5 Cilandro plant as herbal remedy [12].

- *Lemon balm* has a relaxing, antispasmodic effect on the stomach and nervous system. It may help fight off viruses.
- *Peppermint* is a familiar flavor in toothpaste and chewing gum. When brewed as tea, peppermint may relieve digestive discomforts such as indigestion and vomiting.
- *Lavender* is a woody plant that boasts medical benefits as a mild antidepressant. One can add lavender oil to bath to alleviate stress, tension, and insomnia.
- *Cinnamon* has numerous health benefits, and is particularly effective at lowering blood sugar levels. It has potent antioxidant activity, helps fight inflammation, and has been shown to lower cholesterol in the blood.
- *Sage* extract can improve brain and memory function, especially in individuals with Alzheimer's disease.
- *Holy basil* appears to improve immune function and inhibit the growth of bacteria, yeasts, and molds.
- *Cayenne pepper* is a type of chili pepper used to prepare spicy dishes. It has also shown anti-cancer potential in animal studies.
- *Ginger* is an effective treatment for many types of nausea. It is also anti-inflammatory property and can help reduce pain.
- *Fenugreek* can improve the function of insulin, leading to significant reductions in blood sugar levels.
- *Rosemary* has anti-inflammatory effects that appear to suppress allergy symptoms and reduce nasal congestion.

- *Osha* is considered an immune booster and aid for coughs, pneumonia, colds, bronchitis, and the flu.
- *Dill* is a herb that has been shown to have antioxidant, antiprotozoal, antibacterial, and anticancer properties.
- *Aloe* is known for its effectiveness at cooling and soothing sunburn.

Some of these herbs are easy to grow and they bring health benefits to families. They are so ingrained in Mexican culture that they are still used in some parts of Mexico today.

10.5 APPLICATIONS OF MEXICAN TRADITIONAL MEDICINE

The cost of modern medicine is skyrocketing. People face difficulties accessing quality care due to their race or gender and are eager for options outside of the mainstream medical system. Some families who cannot afford modern medicine are turning to more traditional, natural remedies. Today, Mexican indigenous medicinal plants are being used to treat many diseases. Some typical uses of MTM arc described as follows.

- *Fever:* Many regard fever as a disease in and of itself and not as a symptom of a much broader process like infection. The presence of a fever in a young child may be considered by the mother as an emergency situation. Fever is the symptom about which the mother will be most concerned and worrisome [2].
- *Cancer:* Cancer cases are increasing in number worldwide. This makes the disease the second cause of mortality. Medicinal plants have been used in the fight against cancer and today more than 70% of anticancer drugs have a natural origin [14].
- *Diabetes:* This is the most common chronic disease characterized by an increase in glucose levels due to insulin deficiency. The disease is associated with eye, renal, cardiovascular, neurological complications, fatigue, weight loss, delayed wound healing, blurred vision, increases in urine glucose levels, etc. In the absence of proper treatment, cardiac, vascular, neurological, and renal damage may occur. Treatment includes diet, exercise, and medication. Plenty of plants have been investigated for anti–diabetic effects. They can reduce diabetes complications [15].
- *Coronavirus:* Mexican herbalists have gained confidence and good reputations and increased sales of their plants for treatments of respiratory diseases in times of the new coronavirus pandemic. Composed of green tea leaves, chamomile, dandelion, and antiviral make up interferon that help strengthen the immune system [16].
- *Depression and Anxiety:* These are psychiatric disorders, which share similar symptoms. Anxiety is often regarded as a normal reaction to a stressor. Anxiety disorders affect 18% of the general US adult population. People with anxiety disorders often face numerous challenges to take therapy such as a lack of healthcare services. The use of herbal medicine is widespread among those who suffer mood and anxiety disorders. In Mexico, 92 plant species can be used in folk medicine for the treatment of depression and anxiety. For example, chamomile may be clinically relevant due to its antidepressant activity [17].
- *Tuberculosis* (TB): This disease kills about 3 million people per year worldwide. TB is an infectious deadly disease and is associated with individuals suffering from human immunodeficiency virus

(HIV). There is a need for new anti-TB agents. Nine herbal plants have been used in Mexican traditional medicine to treat tuberculosis [18].

- *Diarrhea:* This infectious disease is a great problem throughout the world. It is the cause of considerable morbidity and mortality, especially in developing countries. In Mexico, herbal products are commonly used as therapeutic tools. Traditional medicine uses a great variety of plants in the treatment of diarrhea [19].
- *Obesity:* This is a worldwide medical problem. Obesity is characterized by an increase in the number (hyperplasia) and size (hypertrophy) of adipocytes. It is caused by an increased intake of high-fat diets and physical inactivity. Obesity is one of the major risk factors for type 2 diabetes, cardiovascular disease, hypertension, musculoskeletal diseases, and certain types of cancer. Obesity is a serious health problem and accounts for substantial expenditures in Mexico, which ranks second in the world with respect to the incidence of adult obesity. Antiobesity agents from natural products are gaining attention in the scientific community. New ethnobotanical information regarding the antiobesity effect of medicinal plants has been provided. The consumption of herbal products as a remedy for obesity is harmless because of their natural origin [20].
- *Scorpion Poisoning:* This is a common concern in tropical and subtropical regions, especially in Africa, Latin America, India, and the Middle East. Scorpions present a common risk of poisoning. In Mexico, scorpionism represents a serious public health problem. Mexican traditional herbal plants have been widely used as a remedy for treating scorpion poisoning [21].

Other diseases that have been cured by MTM include skin diseases, fungal infections, foodborne disease, respiratory diseases, and gastrointestinal disorders.

10.6 BENEFITS

Mexico's healthcare system has not been able to meet the needs of its population due to the growing challenges created by the prevalence of noncommunicable diseases such as diabetes, obesity, heart disease, and cancer. People living in rural communities of Mexico have little access to modern healthcare facilities and most of them use traditional medicine. Americans can learn a lot about health from their Mexican neighbors. The adult US population has shown increasing interest in the use of traditional medicine.

Other benefits of MTM include the following:

- *Cost:* Access to medical care is a basic human right. Some people seek options outside of the mainstream medical system. Mexican women perceive herbal remedies as inexpensive, natural, and safe. Some turn to more traditional, natural methods of childbirth, including the use of midwives.
- *Easy-to-grow Medicinal Herbs:* Most folk remedies are harmless. Even novice gardeners can concoct simple home remedies such as teas and salves. This will avoid buying medical herbal products that have longed exposed to light and high temperatures while stored in their plastic containers. You can grow your own herbs to ensure the best quality and potency of your herbal remedies.
- *Availability:* Popular herbs are now readily available at supermarkets, chain health food stores, and fly-by-night sellers, competing with local Mexican herb stores. Popular herbs such as manzanilla are now readily available at supermarkets. There are stores still selling a great variety of herbs in

Chicago, Los Angeles, Amarillo, Oakland, etc. For example, Herbs of Mexico, a shop that was opened in 1961 in Los Angeles, carries herbs that are traditional in Mexican healing practices, It has been registered with the Food and Drug Administration. It does not source herbs whose harvesting is harmful to the environment [10].

- *Biological Diversity:* MTM is regarded for its cultural and biological diversity, which is reflected in the vast traditional knowledge of herbal remedies. Mexico has great biodiversity of fauna, with its common practice since pre-Hispanic times.

10.7 CHALLENGES

Mexican traditional medicine faces some challenges that stem from the renewed interest in herbal medicine. There is also the problem of overdose rates in MTM. While most folk remedies are harmless, some remedies could be potentially fatal. Herbs are not regulated by the Food and Drug Administration (FDA). There is little legal protection. Increased scrutiny and a growing atmosphere of tension and discrimination could deter even documented Latino immigrants from seeking proper care.

Some traditional remedies are potentially fatal. Some of the herbal preparations used to treat selected Mexican-American folk ailments may contain potentially toxic levels of lead. More studies are needed in order to gather information regarding the use of various herbs in México. Making traditional medicine mainstream, incorporating its knowledge into modern healthcare, and ensuring that it meets modern safety and efficacy standards, is an uphill task.

Other challenges faced by MTM include the following [22]:

- *Oral Tradition:* Mexican Traditional Health practitioners passed their knowledge down from generation to generation. These traditional beliefs and practices of healing are still rooted within the many indigenous cultures. Information is transmitted orally, without need for documentation.
- *Safety:* There are concerns about the quality and safety of traditional alternative medical products. Most of these herbal medicines can be purchased directly from health food stores and pharmacies as over-the-counter medications without the proper information. The safety of many of these medicinal plants has not been studied.
- *Interaction:* Some herbs may interact with prescribed medications. This calls for responsible use of TM to avoid interactions with other treatments. Be sure to talk to your healthcare professional or a qualified herbalist before you start taking herbs.
- *MTM Under Threat:* Deforestation, ill-planned urban expansion, uncontrolled livestock grazing, and desertification are currently threatening Mexico's herbal plants. Many indigenous medical plants are being lost or become underappreciated. There is a need to preserve the knowledge of the ancestors, by teaching children how to identify, recognize, protect, and defend medicinal plants. Certain health promoting aspects of Mexican culture are lost as migrants adapt to and adopt American ways of life.
- *Marginalization:* In the US, many Latino immigrant communities, such as indigenous language speakers, are vulnerable and already marginalized from mainstream healthcare services. The growing atmosphere of discrimination could deter these undocumented Latino immigrants from seeking proper care.

- *Regulation:* Some are of the opinion that regulating indigenous medicine in Mexico could violate rights. Efforts to make traditional medicines mainstream have to cope with significant differences in regulation. The Mexican state has proposed legislation that would grant the state authority to regulate and control the practice of indigenous medicine. One goal of the legislation is to curb the activities of people who falsely claim to be traditional healers. The regulation also reduces many fake remedies and false practitioners.
- *Integration:* Combining traditional and modern medicine faces numerous challenges due to key differences in how each is practiced, evaluated, and managed. Integrating traditional medicine into modern healthcare is taken seriously by some of the biggest research bodies worldwide.
- *Legislation:* There is the need of adequate legislation at the state and federal levels to prevent biopiracy and grant recognition to this ancestral wisdom. But traditional medical groups warn against legislation to grant state authority to regulate and control the practice of indigenous medicine. The Mexican state authority also sees the legislation as violating the country's constitution and international conventions on the rights of ancestral communities, academics, and traditional medical groups. It violates the right of self-determination of indigenous communities to preserve their knowledge and cultural identity.
- *Culture Clash:* Dosage of traditional medicine and traditional medicine is varied. Unlike modern drugs, the quality of source material for traditional medicines varies greatly.

Some of these challenges are illustrated in Figure 10.7.

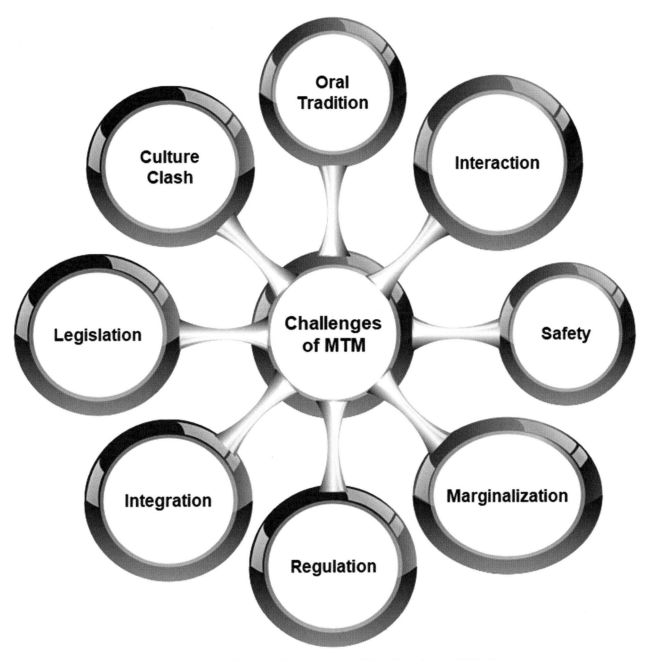

Figure 10.7 Challenges of Mexican traditional medicine (MTM).

10.9 GLOBALIZATION OF MEXICAN MEDICINE

The systematization, documentation, and digitization of the traditional medical knowledge on the traditional medical system of Mexico is very valuable. Traditional Mexican healing practices have survived conquest, colonization, and the professionalization of medicine. It is practiced as a rich tradition by Mexicans, Mexican-Americans, Puerto Ricans, and other Hispanics. Traditional medicine has a lot to offer global health.

To supplement the modern healthcare system, there is a growing interest in traditional medicine both in Mexico and the United States. Traditional or indigenous medicine can bridge some of these barriers to healthcare. The National Autonomous University of Mexico has set up a digital library that lists more than 3,000 indigenous plant species. California School of Herbal Studies was founded in 1978 for herbal education. The Tzu Chi medical team (TIMA) provides a wide range of compassionate healthcare from both Western and alternative medical practices and dental services in Mexico. The team is making enormous impact. They have one big heart — love for all humanity. Figure 10.6 shows the Tzu Chi medical team at work [23].

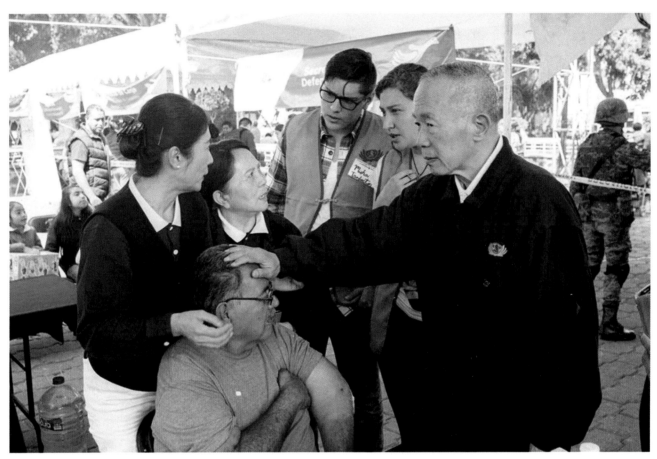

Figure 10.6 The Tzu Chi medical team at work [23].

Recently, it seems that the Mexican Republic has lost the primal connection to the natural world. There is a rising movement to restore ancient plant-based healing practices. Traditional indigenous medicine is recognized in Mexico's constitution as a cultural right. The government of Mexico aims to incorporate and integrate the contributions of traditional indigenous medicine and complementary medicine in the country's healthcare system. The reform vows to recognize, conserve, and protect indigenous medicine in Mexico. This integrative healthcare utilizes techniques such as acupuncture and cupping, a Chinese technique with historical roots in traditional Mexican medicine. Cupping is very safe and very effective.

10.9 CONCLUSION

The traditional medicine industry is worth big money and is rapidly growing. Indigenous people worldwide still reckon with the natural world and safeguard the plant spirits. Many Mexican Americans still practice traditional Mexican medicine due to access to healthcare, cost, and family tradition. For much of humankind, possessing plant knowledge, or being accessible to a person who does, can make the difference between life and death. Regarding MTM as a whole medical practices could help improve health outcomes for Latino patients.

There is a trend to use medicinal plants for primary medical care or as dietary supplements. Scientists are beginning to uncover the efficacy of traditional medicine. It is inevitable that ancient and modern medicines are converging. Integrating traditional medicine into modern system has been taken seriously by some of the biggest research bodies worldwide. Incorporating MTM practices into modern medicine will allow more effective and culturally sensitive healthcare provision for Latino immigrants in the United States. More information about Mexican traditional medicine can be found in the books in [24-42] and the following related journals:

- *Journal of Ethnopharmacology*
- *Journal of Medicinal Plants Research*

REFERENCES

[1] S. C. Guzmán-Rosas et al., "The exclusion of indigenous traditional knowledge in the higher education: The case of traditional medicine and the Mexican medical education," *Creative Education*, vol. 6, 2015, pp. 867-879.

[2] B. Bledsoe, "Understand folk medicine's role in the prehospital care of many Mexican-Americans," November 2009,
https://www.jems.com/training/understand-folk-medicines-role/

[3] "Mexican folk dance images,"
https://www.shutterstock.com/image-photo/guadalajara-mexico-aug-28-participants-parde-498933262

[4] M. S. Geck et al., "Traditional herbal medicine in Mesoamerica: Toward its evidence base for improving universal health coverage," *Frontiers in Pharmacology*, July 2020.

[5] M. N. O. Sadiku, G. K. Suman, and S. M. Musa, "Mexican traditional medicine: A primer," *International Journal of Trend in Research and Development*, vol. 9, no. 1, January-February 2022, pp. 41-44.

[6] "Folk medicine and traditional healing,"
http://www.ncfh.org/uploads/3/8/6/8/38685499/folk_medicine_and_traditional_healing.pdf

[7] S. G. Marshall, "The childbearing beliefs and practices of pregnant Mexican American adolescents living in southwest border regions," *Masters Thesis*, University of Arizona, 1987.

[8] A. Joyce, "The sixth sun: The spiritual path and practice of Mexican-American curanderismo," *Doctoral Dissertation*, California Institute of Integral Studies, 2011.

[9] J. G. Gladstein, " Mexico's alternative medicine in Amarillo, Texas,"
https://www.mexconnect.com/articles/3661-mexico-s-alternative-medicine-in-amarillo-texas/

[10] "Meet Mexico's curandero healers keeping indigenous culture alive,"
https://theculturetrip.com/north-america/mexico/articles/meet-mexicos-curandero-healers-enacting-surgical-miracles/

[11] "Herbs of Mexico, supplying authentic home remedies for the people of east Los Angeles for more than 50 years,"

https://www.lataco.com/herbs-of-mexico-authentic-home-remedies-store-east-la/

[12] "Homegrown herbal remedies,"
https://www.healthline.com/health/herbal-remedies-from-your-garden

[13] "Medicinal plants: Sold at traditional Mexican markets,"
https://www.backyardnature.net/m/produce/mediherb.htm

[14] N. J. Jacobo-Herrera et al., "Medicinal plants used in Mexican traditional medicine for the treatment of colorectal cancer," *Journal of Ethnopharmacology,* vol. 179, February 2016, pp. 391-402.

[15] B. Moradi et al., "The most useful medicinal herbs to treat diabetes," *The Vietnamese Journal of Biomedicine*, vol 5, no 8, 2018, pp. 2538-2551.

[16] "Coronavirus marks the rebirth of traditional medicine in Mexico," April 2020,
https://www.archyde.com/coronavirus-marks-the-rebirth-of-traditional-medicine-in-mexico/

[17] S. L. G. Gutiérreza, R. R. Chilpab, and H. B. Jaimea, "Medicinal plants for the treatment of 'nervios', anxiety, and depression in Mexican traditional medicine*," Revista Brasileira de Farmacognosia*, vol. 24, 2014, pp. 591-608.

[18] M. R. Camacho-Corona et al., "Activity against drug resistant-tuberculosis strains of plants used in Mexican traditional medicine to treat tuberculosis and other respiratory diseases," *Phytotherapy Research*, vol. 22, 2008, pp. 82-85.

[19] E. Barbosa, F. Calzada, and R. Campos, "In vivo antigiardial activity of three flavonoids isolated of some medicinal plants used in Mexican traditional medicine for the treatment of diarrhea," *Journal of Ethnopharmacology*, vol. 109, 2007, pp. 552–554.

[20] A. J. Alonso-Castro et al., "Plants used in the traditional medicine of Mesoamerica (Mexico and Central America) and the Caribbean for the treatment of obesity," *Journal of Ethnopharmacology*, vol. 175, December 2015, pp. 335-345.

[21] J. E. Jime´nez-Ferrera, "Antitoxin activity of plants used in Mexican traditional medicine against scorpion poisoning," *Phytomedicine*, vol. 12, 2005, pp. 116–122.

[22] "Regulating indigenous medicine in Mexico 'could violate rights',"
https://news.knowledia.com/CA/en/articles/regulating-indigenous-medicine-in-mexico-could-violate-rights-3083d788f2d75901dd9ab35ffb2c23ded94188bc

[23] "Mexico medical mission: Compassionate healthcare through integrative medicine," April 2019,
https://tzuchimedical.us/blog/mexico-medical-mission-compassionate-healthcare-through-integrative-medicine

[24] C. E. Flores, *Exploring Traditional Herbal Remedies in Mexico: An Introduction to Natural Healing.* Kindle Edition, 2020.

[25] C. Flores, *The Mexican Apothecary: Traditional Cold and Flu Herbal Remedies.* ndependently Published, 2019.

[26] A. DeStefano, *Latino Folk Medicine: Healing Herbal Remedies from Ancient Traditions.* Ballantine Books, 2001.

[27] E. Torres, *Green Medicine: Traditional Mexican-American Herbal Remedies.* Nieves Press, 1983.

[28] J. Davidow, *Infusions of Healing: A Treasury of Mexican-American Herbal Remedies.* Atria Books, 1999.

[29] A. Sandoval, *Homegrown Healing: Traditional Home Remedies From Mexico Mass Market.* Berkley, 1998.

[30] A. Chevallier, *Encyclopedia of Herbal Medicine: 550 Herbs and Remedies for Common Ailments.* DK, 3rd edition, 2016.

[31] J. O. West, *Mexican-American Folklore.* August House Publishers, 2005.

[32] R. T. Trotter II and J. A. Chavira, *Curanderismo: Mexican American Folk Healing*. University of Georgia Press, 2nd edition, 1997.

[33] F. Altamirano, *Materia Medica Mexicana - A Manual of Mexican Medicinal Herbs*. Deutsch Press, 2011.

[34] G. Schendel, *Medicine in Mexico. From Aztec Herbs to Betatrons*. University of Texas Press, Austin, TX, 1968.

[35] A.V. Ellis, *Letras y Limpias: Decolonial Medicine and Holistic Healing in Mexican American Literature*. University of Arizona Press, 2021.

[36] E. Torres, *The Folk Healer: The Mexican-American Tradition of Curanderismo*. Nieves Press, 2021.

[37] J. Davidow, *Infusions of Healing: A Treasury of Mexican-American Herbal Remedies*. Fireside, 1999.

[38] *Herbolaria Mexicana: Encyclopedia Medicinal (Spanish Edition)*. Hawthorne, CA: GF Books, 2017.

[39] E. Torres and I. Miranda, *Curandero: Traditional Healers of Mexico and the Southwest*. Kendall Hunt Publishing, 2017.

[40] E. Torres, *Curanderismo: The Art of Traditional Medicine without Borders*. Kendall Hunt Publishing, 2017.

[41] S. Chavez-Hilton, *Curanderismo Healing: Mind Body and Spirit: Indigenous Wellness Series: Healing Ceremonies*. Estara Health, 2015.

[42] M. Silva, *Curanderismo: The Ultimate Guide to Latin American Folk Healing and Shamanism (Spiritual Healing)*. Independently published, 2022.

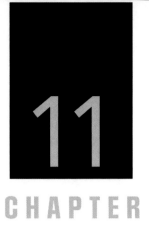

Traditional Mediterranean Diet

"It is a very brave choice to go against traditional medicine and embrace the alternative route. It's easier to try the traditional route and then, if it fails, go to the alternatives, but often it can be too late." - Suzanne Somers

11.1 INTRODUCTION

The modernization and globalization of the world's diet has resulted in various diseases that now seem linked to the modern age: cardiovascular disease, diabetes, cancer, and obesity. The traditional system of medicine is used in various part of the globe. Interest in the traditional diet began in the 1950s when it was noted that heart disease was not as common in Mediterranean countries as it was in the US. All regions have their own unique traditional diets: Latin America, Africa, Asia, the Arctic, and Europe. A dietary data from the Mediterranean region show that in the recent past the inhabitants of this region enjoy the lowest recorded rates of chronic diseases and the highest adult life expectancy due to their eating pattern. This has made Mediterranean diet to be widely recognized as one of the healthiest diets in the world.

Traditional Mediterranean diet (MedDiet) is the old way of eating. It is one of the most studied and well-known dietary models worldwide. It is a delicious and pleasant roadmap to healthy eating and happy living. The Mediterranean diet has been characterized as the gold standard of diets. It is a lifestyle approach to eating rooted in a centuries-old tradition of using fresh, high-quality ingredients. It features foods grown all around the Mediterranean Sea. It is a pattern of eating that is modeled after the traditional cuisines of people living in certain regions bordering the Mediterranean Sea. There are 21 nations that touch the Mediterranean Sea: Albania, Algeria, Bosnia and Herzegovina, Croatia, Cyprus, Egypt, France, Greece, Israel, Italy, Lebanon, Libya, Malta, Monaco, Montenegro, Morocco, Slovenia, Spain, Syria, Tunisia, and Turkey, all areas where food is prepared to be savored and enjoyed, not rushed [1]. Figure 11.1 shows the Mediterranean sea with the surrounding countries [2]. Although the diet varies by country and region due to differences in culture, ethnic background, religion, economy, geography, and agricultural production. The Mediterranean approach to eating regards food as a communal, shared experience. It is a way of eating rather than a formal diet plan.

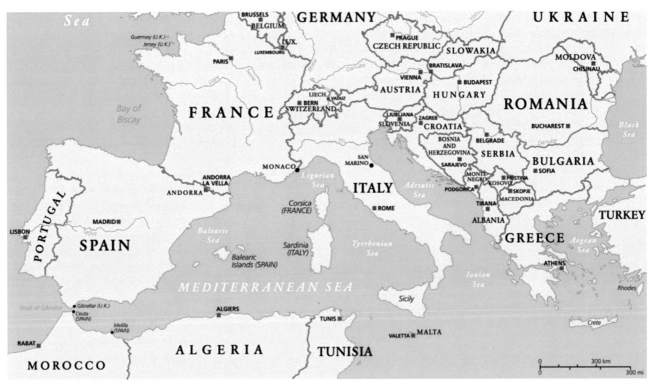

Figure 11.1 The Mediterranean sea and the surrounding countries [2].

The Mediterranean diet is a healthy-eating plan that incorporates the traditional flavors and cooking methods of the region. The traditional Mediterranean diet is characterized by a high intake of vegetables, legumes, fruits and nuts, and cereals with a high intake of olive oil, a moderately high intake of fish, a low intake of meat and poultry, and a moderate intake of wine. A healthy diet can improve your ability to think, improve heart health, enhance brain health, and lower risk of dementia [3,4].

This chapter provides an introduction to Mediterranean herbs or diet. It begins by providing a brief history about the traditional Mediterranean diet (MedDiet). It presents some popular Mediterranean herbs and vegetables. It covers the standard Mediterranean diet as well as other types of Mediterranean diet. It discusses some applications of MedDiet. It highlights the benefits and challenges of MedDiet. It explains globalization of MedDiet. The last section concludes with comments.

11.2 BRIEF HISTORY OF MEDITARIAN DIET

Written history allows tracing back Mediterranean and European medical traditions to Greek antiquity. The cultivation and use of vegetables, herbs, and spices in the Eastern region of the Mediterranean date back to the ancient Egyptian, Greek, and Roman civilizations. The ancient Mediterranean region was rich in vibrant colors, flavors, and remedies that helped keep the civilizations of Greece, Rome, and Egypt thriving for thousands of years.

Interest in the diet began in the 1950s when it was noted that heart disease was not as common in Mediterranean countries as it was in the US. Since then, numerous studies have confirmed that the Mediterranean diet helps prevent heart disease and stroke. In 1948, the first ever study of the now known Mediterranean diet happened in Crete. In 1948 the Greek government invited the Rockefeller foundation to investigate how to raise the standard of living in post war Crete. The study was very thorough and it was discovered that the diet of the Cretans was nutritionally adequate compared to the US nutrition standards. The typical dietary pattern of Crete in the 50's and 60's was associated with good health and the lowest rates of heart disease [5].

From 1952–1957, American researcher Ancel Keys conducted exploratory studies in seven countries: Italy, Greece, Yugoslavia, the Netherlands, Finland, Japan, and the United States. Keys and his collaborators concluded that dietary patterns in Italy and Greece were associated with the lower rates of heart disease and all-cause mortality in these countries [1]. In 1993, the Mediterranean Diet Food pyramid was developed by researchers and WHO. In essence, it was the introduction of the Mediterranean diet to the American public. In 2000 and beyond, the Mediterranean diet goes mainstream. The Mediterranean diet began gaining momentum particularly after the fat phobia of the 90's. Year after year, the Mediterranean diet comes out on top in the US News and World Report annual ranking of best diets.

11.3 MEDITERRANEAN HERBS

Traditionally, herbs refer to leafy parts of plants, while spices is generally adopted for preparations from roots, seeds, root bark, berries, flower parts, fruits, or other plant parts. There is a wide variety of herbs colors, shapes, sizes, and flowering available. Herbal medicines are culturally accepted and widely used in many nations for treating a variety of disorders. Popular Mediterranean herbs and vegetables include the following [6,7]:

- *Rosemary* is a perennial plant whose extracts are used routinely for cooking, preservation of foods, cosmetics, nervous issues, headaches, digestive troubles, female complaints, and herbal medicine for anti-inflammatory and antimicrobial applications. It is native to warmer climates.
- *Licorice* may be used in treating gastric and duodenal ulcers as it reduces stomach secretions and produces protective mucus for the lining of the digestive tract.
- *Helichrysum italicum* is viewed as the sleeping giant of Mediterranean herbal medicine. The use of its essential oil in glamorous perfumes, personal care products, and reducing scars has turned it into a veritable icon of luxury. Today, there is a huge disconnect between demand and availability of the herb. Its flowers are often used to make herbal tea.
- *Basil* is popular known as an Italian spice, shown in Figure 11.2 [7]. Traditional folk medicine in India hails basil as a stress-relieving herb, helpful for those with asthma, and supportive for those with Type 2 diabetes.

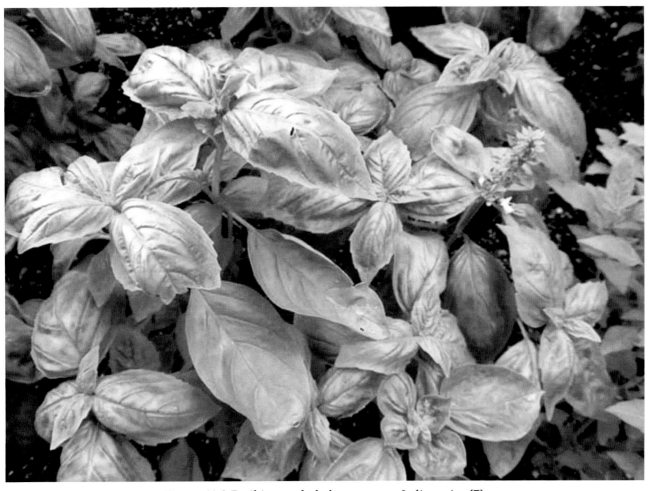

Figure 11.2 Basil is popularly known as an Italian spice [7].

- *Oregano* is a fragrant and aromatic herb, native to the Mediterranean region. Before the age of modern medicine in Europe, oregano was used for digestive, respiratory, nervous, and hormonal complaints.
- *Sage* is practically used for food preservation like rosemary. The herb is reputed as "cure-all," in that it could heal any illness or disease. Most herbalists observe its effectiveness in cases of cold, flu, fever, female issues, and digestive troubles.
- *Thyme* is a powerful plant that is native to the Mediterranean region. Traditional herbalists claim that thyme has the abilities to heal infections, colds, flu, and women's complaints. It was also known to support labor, pregnancy, and gestive issues.

11.4 MEDITERRANEAN DIET

The term Mediterranean diet (MedDiet) was coined by the American scientist Ancel keys in 1960. It is essentially the traditional foods that people used to eat in nations bordering the Mediterranean Sea including France, Spain, Greece, and Italy. It has been observed that these people were exceptionally healthy and had a low risk of many chronic conditions. The diet emphasizes plant-based foods such as vegetables, beans, whole grain, fruits, nuts and seeds, and olive oil and fish. These foods make up the base of the Mediterranean food pyramid, shown in Figure 11.3 [8]. The Mediterranean diet food pyramid reprioritizes the traditional food pyramid. Three factors hold true throughout the Mediterranean region [9]:

1. Food is treated as medicine.
2. Moderation is key.
3. An active physical and social lifestyle is mandatory.

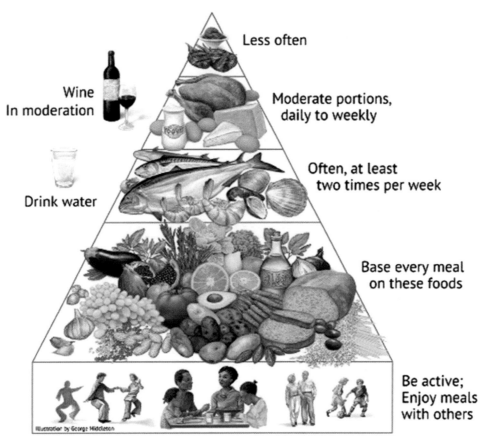

Figure 11.3 The Mediterranean diet pyramid [8].

The Mediterranean diet has become popular because of its association in Mediterranean populations with reduced incidence of some chronic diseases including cancer, coronary heart disease, and cardiovascular disease.

There are many types of Mediterranean diets. A typical Mediterranean one is depicted in Figure 11.4 [10]. The Mediterranean diet does not have preservatives. It is freshly plucked and cooked. The diet encourages fruits, vegetables, whole grains, legumes, nuts, seeds, and heart-healthy fats. So one should base diet on the following healthy Mediterranean foods [11]:

- Vegetables: tomatoes, broccoli, *kale*, spinach, onions, cauliflower, carrots, Brussels sprouts, cucumbers, potatoes, sweet potatoes, turnips
- Fruits: apples, bananas, oranges, pears, strawberries, grapes, *dates*, figs, melons, peaches
- Nuts, seeds, and nut butters: almonds, *walnuts*, macadamia nuts, hazelnuts, cashews, sunflower seeds, pumpkin seeds, almond butter, peanut butter
- Legumes: beans, peas, lentils, pulses, peanuts, chickpeas
- Whole grains: oats, brown rice, rye, barley, corn, buckwheat, whole wheat bread and pasta

- Fish and seafood: *salmon*, sardines, trout, tuna, mackerel, shrimp, oysters, clams, crab, mussels
- Poultry: chicken, duck, turkey
- Eggs: chicken, quail, and duck eggs
- Dairy: cheese, yogurt, milk
- Herbs and spices: *garlic,* basil, mint, rosemary, sage, nutmeg, cinnamon, pepper
- Healthy fats: extra virgin olive oil, olives, *avocados,* and *avocado oil*

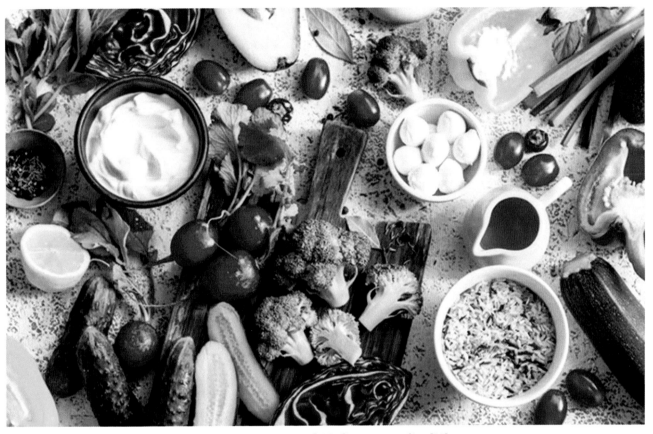

Figure 11.4 A typical Mediterranean diet [10].

Olive oil is very important in Mediterranean diet. It has been used for centuries in Greece and other Mediterranean nations for its beneficial health properties. Olive oil is extracted from the fruit. Application of olive oil with honey has been shown to be effective in a number of skin and fungal infections. There is a strong correlation between olive oil consumption and reduced hypertension. The Food and Drug Administration in US has recommended that two teaspoonfuls of olive oil (23 g) per day. Extra virgin olive oil is used for cooking purposed including roasting, sautéing, and baking [12].

Eating pattern that incorporates these foods promotes good health and weight control. The diet discourages processed foods, added sugar, and refined grains. So one should avoid or limit the following processed foods and ingredients when following the Mediterranean diet:

- Added sugar: *added sugar* is found in many foods but especially high in soda, candies, ice cream, table sugar, syrup, and baked goods
- Refined grains: white bread, pasta, tortillas, chips, crackers
- Trans fats: found in *margarine,* fried foods, and other processed foods

- Refined oils: soybean oil, *canola oil*, cottonseed oil, grapeseed oil
- Processed meat: processed sausages, hot dogs, deli meats, beef jerky
- Highly processed foods: fast food, convenience meals, microwave popcorn, granola bars

There are many ways of incorporating Mediterranean diet into your daily menu. Below is a typical sample menu for 1 week of meals on the Mediterranean diet [11]:

Monday

- Breakfast: Greek yogurt with strawberries and chia seeds
- Lunch: a *whole grain* sandwich with hummus and vegetables
- Dinner: a tuna salad with greens and olive oil, as well as a fruit salad

Tuesday

- Breakfast: oatmeal with blueberries
- Lunch: caprese zucchini noodles with mozzarella, cherry tomatoes, olive oil, and balsamic vinegar
- Dinner: a salad with tomatoes, olives, cucumbers, farro, grilled chicken, and feta cheese

Wednesday

- Breakfast: an omelet with mushrooms, tomatoes, and onions
- Lunch: a whole grain sandwich with cheese and fresh vegetables
- Dinner: Mediterranean lasagna

Thursday

- Breakfast: *yogurt* with sliced fruit and nuts
- Lunch: a quinoa salad with chickpeas
- Dinner: broiled salmon with brown rice and vegetables

Friday

- Breakfast: eggs and sautéed vegetables with whole wheat toast
- Lunch: stuffed zucchini boats with pesto, turkey sausage, tomatoes, bell peppers, and cheese
- Dinner: grilled lamb with salad and baked potato

Saturday

- Breakfast: oatmeal with raisins, nuts, and apple slices
- Lunch: a whole grain sandwich with vegetables
- Dinner: Mediterranean pizza made with whole wheat pita bread and topped with cheese, vegetables, and olives

Sunday

- Breakfast: an omelet with veggies and olives
- Lunch: falafel bowl with feta, onions, tomatoes, hummus, and rice
- Dinner: grilled chicken with vegetables, sweet potato fries, and fresh fruit

One can adapt the portions and food choices recommended above in a way that works for you.

11.5 OTHER TYPES OF MEDITERRANEAN DIETS

There are many types of Mediterranean diets because the diet varies by region and nation. Mediterranean diet is a generic term for traditional diet of nations bordering the Mediterranean Sea and there is no one standard Mediterranean diet. 21 nations border the Mediterranean. Eating styles vary among the nations due to differences in culture, ethnic background, religion, economy, geography, and agricultural production. Variations of the MedDiet exist in Italy, France, Lebanon, Morocco, Portugal, Spain, Tunisia, Turkey, and elsewhere in the Mediterranean region. So many of the diets across the Mediterranean are not consistent with the Mediterranean diet pattern even within the same country.

- *Nordic Diet*: The Nordic diet is similar to the Mediterranean diet except that it emphasizes canola oil instead of extra virgin olive oil. This incorporates foods commonly eaten by people in the Nordic countries: Norway, Denmark, Sweden, Finland, and Iceland. It was created in 2004 by a team of nutritionists, scientists, and chefs to address growing obesity rates and unsustainable farming practices in the Nordic countries. It replaces processed foods with whole, single-ingredient ones [13].
- *Diet of Crete:* The traditional diet of Crete in Greece has the lowest rates of heart disease, all-cause mortality, and cancer. The diet is based on traditional agricultural practices and utilization of natural resources. There are components of the traditional diet of Crete that are not included in "the Mediterranean diet." There are also lifestyle factors that have been shown to independently provide health benefits [14].
- *Diet of Greece:* Multipurpose herbal teas with numerous ingredients are common in the traditional medicine and pharmacy of Greece. Flowers are the main component of the ingredients. These blends are consumed for their relaxing, digestive, and anti-infective properties. These mixtures are for preventive measure. The flowers of Rosaceae, Asteraceae, Lamiaceae, Malvaceae, and Fabaceae species characterize these mixtures in which other materials (roots, leaves, and fruits) and other species [15].
- *Diet of Algeria:* In Algeria, phytotherapy is an important component of the local culture of population which holds an important knowledge acquired empirically from a generation to another. Indeed, Algeria is characterized by a very rich and highly diversified flora. The use of aromatic and medicinal plants and their derivatives for food and therapeutic purposes is common in the region of Tiaret (Algeria). Herbalists prescribe most of their preparations through oral administration. The recommend the use of mixtures based on several plant species with other ingredients such as honey, olive oil, goat milk and butter, water, yogurt, eggs, etc. to improve the taste and enhance the therapeutic effects [16].

- *Diet of Syria:* Syria is one of the countries in the Mediterranean area with climatic condition that is conducive for the development of varied vegetation and plant species. Syrians have excellent medical knowledge and traditional experience of basic medicinal plants. Some plants may have dual antiviral and immunomodulating effects, and thus can be adopted in preventing the spread of COVID-19, which can affect both animals and humans. People with these symptoms may have COVID-19: fever or chills, cough, shortness of breath or difficulty breathing, fatigue, muscle or body aches, headache, new loss of taste or smell, sore throat, congestion or runny nose, nausea or vomiting, diarrhea [17].

- *Diet of Turkey:* This region is blessed with a rich flora, providing a rich tradition of folk medicine based on medicinal plants. A large proportion of these plants is used to treat gastrointestinal disorders. This probably is the result of the habit of eating spicy foods in the region. These plants are usually employed in the liquid form (decoction, infusion). Sometimes they are eaten either fresh or dried. Knowledge of the use of plants as remedies is apparently the result of transmission from the old to the new generation. Turkish native herbs from both natural and cultivated sources are being more widely used on a commercial scale in the food industry, in traditional medicine, and for their flavoring properties [18,19].

11.6 APPLICATIONS OF MEDITERRANEAN DIET

Mediterranean diet is generally rich in healthy plant foods and relatively lower in animal foods, with a focus on fish and seafood. The diet is healthier than modern ones that have processed foods and sugar. Doctors and dietitians recommend a Mediterranean diet to prevent disease and keep people healthy for longer. As shown in Figure 11.5, Harvard Medical School has a handy graphic that can help you build your meals based on Mediterannean-friendly foods [20]. Taking a Mediterranean diet may reduce the risk of muscle weakness in older age, Alzheimer's disease, Parkinson's disease, and premature death. Mediterranean diet has an almost limitless ability to provide healing to many diseases, as demonstrated by the following examples.

- *Osteoarthritis:* This is the most common form of arthritis, affecting thousands of people. The condition is often noticed it in the knees, hands, hips, or spine. Making changes to your diet can help you with osteoarthritis symptoms, which include pain, stiffness, and swelling. Taking a balanced, nutritious diet will improve osteoarthritis and give the body the tools it needs to prevent further damage to the joints [21].

- *Longevity:* Following traditional Mediterranean diet promotes longevity. A person who follows the Mediterranean diet will live longer, even if he does not live in the Mediterranean region. The traditional Mediterranean diet features an abundance of vegetables, legumes, fruits, nuts, and cereals and regular use of olive oil. Researchers have observed that those who strongly adhere to a Mediterranean diet had improved longevity compared to study participants who did not follow that diet as closely [22]. The Mediterranean diet has been shown to be protective against chronic disease, and increase longevity according to numerous clinical studies.

- *Cancer:* The traditional Mediterranean diet is rich in substances that have protective effects such as selenium, vitamin E and C, omega-3 fatty acids, fiber, antioxidants from herbs such as oregano and garlic. These nutrients are associated with a lower risk of cancer, particularly prostate, breast, and colon cancer [5]. Recent studies provide evidence that greater adherence to the Mediterranean diet is inversely associated with cancer mortality in the general population, hence increased longevity. Regular intake of Mediterranean diet can reduce the risk of cancers including breast cancer, ovarian cancer, urinary tract cancer, gastrointestinal cancers, etc.

- *Diabetes*: This disease has reached epidemic proportions and is at the forefront of public health problems, affecting 451 million people worldwide in 2017. Following a healthful eating pattern, such as the Mediterranean eating plan, is an effective way to manage type 2 diabetes [23].

- *Overweight and Obesity:* Being overweight or obese places extra pressure on the joints. A poor diet is a common reason people struggle with weight loss. The Mediterranean diet plan has become one of the most recommended diets for weight loss and disease prevention. It is ideal for weight loss compared to a Westernized diet. The Mediterranean diet is helpful for people who are trying to lose weight. It helps a person to lose weight and keep it off. The Mediterranean diet not only reduces body weight, it also reduces waist circumference and body mass index [24].

- *Cardiovascular Disease:* Several studies have been conducted to evaluate the effects of Mediterranean diet on CVD outcomes, including blood lipids, blood pressure, inflammatory biomarkers, and body weight. Recent studies have shown the benefits of the Mediterranean diet on cardiovascular health, including reduction in the incidence of cardiovascular disease. The Primary Prevention of Cardiovascular Disease with a Mediterranean Diet (PREDIMED) study (published in the New England Journal of Medicine) is the largest intervention study and one of the most well-known studies to examine the effects of the Mediterranean diet on cardiovascular prevention among persons at high risk of CVD [25].

- *Pregnancy*: This is one of the difficult periods in the life of a woman. Her body undergoes may change and the diet followed can make a big difference in her health and that of the fetus. Mediterranean diet, being a balanced dietary pattern, may ensure a smooth progression and contribute to a healthy weight of the expected mother during pregnancy. Many studies have highlighted the protective role of the Mediterranean diet against the occurrence of gestational diabetes and hypertension during pregnancy [26].

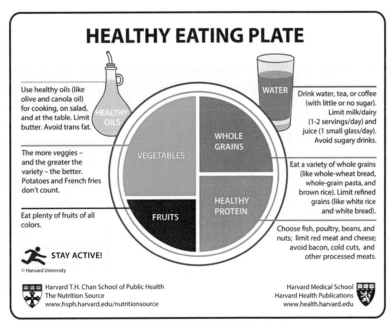

Figure 11.5 Harvard Medical School has a handy graphic for Mediterranean-friendly foods [20].

11.7 BENEFITS

The benefits of the Mediterranean diet are ever increasing. It is known as one of the healthiest in the world because it is not just a diet, but a lifestyle that is based on a variety of healthy foods. The Mediterranean diet has received much attention as a healthy way of eating. It comes out on top in the US News and World Report ranking of best diets in 2021, 2020, 2019, and 2018. Mediterranean herbs are of great importance as a mechanism to increase access to health care services.

Other benefits of a Mediterranean diet include [5]:

- *Simple Diet:* The eating the Mediterranean way is flexible, healthy, cheap, easy to follow, and backed by research and experience. Following a Mediterranean diet might be a good thing to do for your health. Thousands of people who follow eating Mediterranean-style could lower risk for chronic diseases. This diet can help one maintain a healthy weight without counting calories, or following complicated rules.
- *Staying Healthy:* Eating a balanced diet will help one to stay healthy. It provides all the nutrients a person requires and avoids eating junk food. Mediterranean diet may help protect brain function, promote heart health, and regulate blood sugar levels. It has long been seen as a healthy way of lowering the risk of heart disease and leading a healthier life.
- *Brain Health:* The Mediterranean diet might help promote and prolong healthy brain function. It could delay the onset of Alzheimer's by up to 3.5 years when compared to people who follow a Western diet. Figure 11.6 shows the importance of the Mediterranean dietary and lifestyle for the protection of brain health.

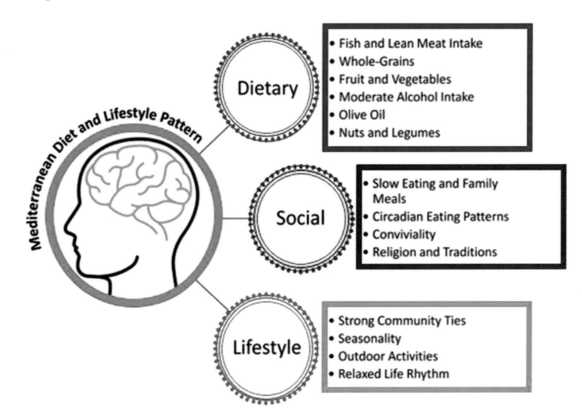

Figure 11.6 The importance of the Mediterranean dietary and lifestyle for the protection of brain health.

- *Preventing Diseases*: Taking a Mediterranean diet can prevent heart disease and stroke and reduce risk factors such as obesity, diabetes, high cholesterol, and high blood pressure. For example, a Mediterranean diet with olive oil or nuts may reduce the combined risk of stroke, heart attack, and death from heart disease. People who follow the Mediterranean diet experience reductions in bad cholesterol, along with improvements in several other heart disease risk factor.

- *Heart Health:* The Mediterranean is well known for its ability to promote heart health. The diet can reduce the risk of cardiovascular disease and stroke. It is a healthy way of lowering the risk of heart disease and leading a healthier life. This is likely due to the fact that following a Mediterannean diet can reduce inflammation in the blood vessels that lead to and from the heart.

- *Improving Sleep Quality:* Research has shown that adhering to a Mediterranean diet may improve sleep quality in older adults. The diet did not seem to affect sleep quality in younger people.

- *Alzheimer's Protection:* Mediterranean diet can reduce the risk of cognitive decline that may appear during the aging process. It can slow some changes in the brain that may point to early Alzheimer's disease.

- *Weight Loss:* A poor diet is a major reason people struggle with weight loss. Adherence to the Mediterranean diet reduces overweight and obesity.

- *Diabetes*: Following a Mediterranean diet can help people with diabetes better control their blood sugar levels. For those with diabetes, the American Diabetes Association recommends eating about less than 20 grams of saturated fat per day.

- *Longevity:* Adherence to the Mediterranean diet has been associated with a reduction in total mortality. The Mediterranean diet has been shown to be protective against chronic disease, cancer, all cause mortality, and increase longevity. Following the Mediterranean diet causes high life expectancy, even if one does not live in a nation in the Mediterranean region.

- *Low Environmental Impacts*: The MedDiet has relatively low environmental impacts (water, nitrogen and carbon footprint). It has been proposed as a "gold standard" diet due to its major health and nutrition benefits. It also has lower environmental impact. The typical food produced in Mediterranean regions and exported/imported from other regions has limited environmental impacts.

Some of these benefits are shown in Figure 11.7.

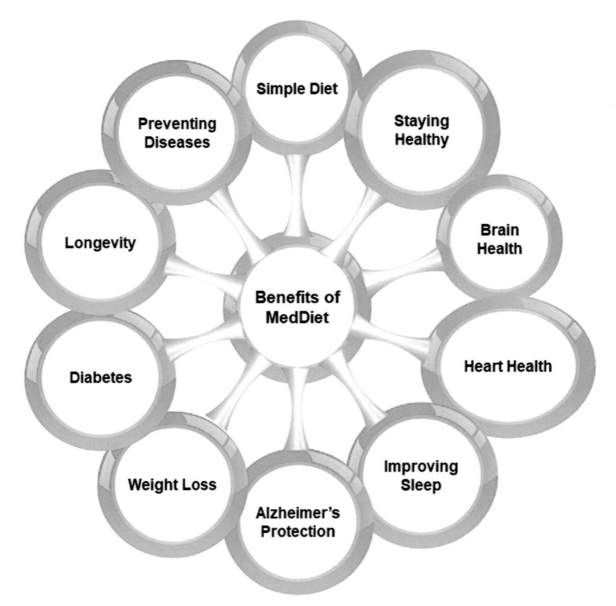

Figure 11.7 Benefits of traditional Mediterranean diet (MedDiet).

11.8 CHALLENGES

The main drawbacks of MedDiet may involve cooking more than you are accustomed to and it may mean adapting to new foods. Although the health benefits mentioned above are indeed real, they are only for those who can pay. People with higher socioeconomic position (higher income, or greater educational level) demonstrate more favorable eating behaviors. We need to guarantee equal access to Mediterranean diet.

Most Mediterranean diet meal plans are not authentic. Even health experts do not agree on the detail of the Mediterranean diet. The diet involves a set of skills, knowledge, rituals, and particularly the consumption of food. It is based on a rural lifestyle, which is fast disappearing [28]. Medicinal plants in the Eastern region of the Mediterranean and other regions are becoming increasingly rare due to the ongoing destruction of their natural habitat, overharvesting of wild species, and detrimental climatic and environmental changes. The UN has recognized the diet as an endangered species [29].

In some cases, herbs used today may not even correspond to the plants described originally in the old literature, as the former are cultivated from herbs that went through different breeding procedures throughout several centuries.

11.9 GLOBALIZATION OF MEDITERRANEAN DIET

In the last few decades, the Western world has moved away from home-grown fresh foods (slow food) to a diet of mass produced, highly processed foods (fast food). The modernization and globalization of food production and processing has resulted in various diseases such as cardiovascular disease, diabetes, cancer, and obesity [30].

The Mediterranean diet is one of the most studied and well-known dietary patterns worldwide. It has drawn lots of praise for its health benefits in ways that a standard Western diet cannot. It is a traditional eating lifestyle that offers flexibility to incorporate a wide range of nutrient-dense foods. Its tenets include eating plenty of plants, low-fat dairy, high fiber foods, and whole grains. This eating pattern is flexible enough to fit many eating traditions around the world. The MedDiet is a sustainable lifestyle model that could likely be followed in other regions and nations. The combination of a healthy diet with social behaviors and the way of life of Mediterranean regions makes the MedDiet a sustainable lifestyle model for other regions.

Although the Mediterranean diet was initially studied in nations around the Mediterranean Sea, the benefits of the healthy diet can be generalizable to many nations such the United States, Canada, Australia, and the United Kingdom. Globalization and advances in food industry have transformed the traditional Mediterranean diet of most Mediterranean regions into a more global dietary patterns. Since food systems are a major cause of poor health, global efforts are urgently needed to collectively transform diets and food production. Public health policies to promote Mediterranean diet at different levels (schools, universities, clinics, hospitals, etc.) should be a cornerstone for the prevention of chronic disease at the national and international levels [31].

The year 2020 celebrated the tenth anniversary of the recognition of the Mediterranean Diet as Intangible Cultural Heritage of Humanity by the UNESCO Intergovernmental Committee. This event was a milestone in the history of traditional diet and the Mediterranean diet was the first traditional food practice to receive such award [32].

Up till now, no effective and accepted tool has been available to monitor the global use of TCAM, and particularly in the Mediterranean. It is particularly effective in solving certain cultural health problems. It is accessible and affordable in rural areas while the chemical drugs are not. Following a Mediterranean diet is proven to lower bad cholesterol, dramatically reduce the risk of heart disease, and may even protect brain function at old age.

11.10 CONCLUSION

Traditional diets represent an expression of people's culture and lifestyle, and a reflection of the region's history, geography, climate, and agriculture. The nations bordering the Mediterranean Sea have long been known for their simple, relaxed, delicious, and family-oriented approach to mealtime. The Mediterranean diet nourishes your body, your heart, and your soul. It appears to improve various risk factors for heart disease. It can be viewed as a way of life. It is gaining an increasing importance in the management of various ailments. The Mediterranean diet is easily adaptable into today's busy lifestyle and suitable for modern palates.

Beyond the diet, the Mediterranean lifestyle encourages mindfulness with every meal.

More information about Mediterranean diet can be found in the books in [33-50] and the following related journals:

- *Journal of Herbal Medicine*
- *Journal of Ethnopharmacology.*
- *Chinese Journal of Integrative Medicine*
- *The Development of Nutraceuticals and Traditional Medicine*
- *Journal of Ethnobiology and Ethnomedicine*
- *Mediterranean Botany*

REFERENCES

[1]   "The problem with the Mediterranean diet we're not talking about enough," https://www.healthline.com/nutrition/the-problem-with-the-mediterranean-diet-were-not-talking-about-enough

[2]   M. Raynor, "The Mediterranean sea could disappear in the distant future," August 2018, https://www.mentalfloss.com/article/555882/mediterranean-sea-could-disappear-distant-future

[3]   A. Trichopoulou et al., "Adherence to a Mediterranean diet and survival in a Greek population," June 2003, https://www.nejm.org/doi/full/10.1056/nejmoa025039

[4]   M. N. O. Sadiku, U. C. Chukwu, A. Ajayi-Majebi, S. M. Musa, "Mediterranean traditional medicine," *International Journal of Trend in Scientific Research and Development,* vol. 6, no. 1, November-December 2021, pp.1206-1213.

[5]   E. Paravantes, "The complete guide to the authentic Mediterranean diet," https://www.olivetomato.com/complete-guide-authentic-mediterranean-diet/

[6]   S. C. Degner, A. J. Papoutsis, and D. F. Romagnolo, "Health benefits of traditional culinary and medicinal Mediterranean plants," *Complementary and Alternative Therapies and the Aging Population,* 2009, 541–562.

[7]   A. White, "The top 5 Mediterranean herbs: Growing, eating, and healing," May 2021. https://gardenerspath.com/plants/herbs/the-top-5-mediterranean-herbs/

[8]   "Mediterranean diet 101 brochure," https://oldwayspt.org/resources/mediterranean-diet-101-brochure

[9]   A. Riolo, "Defining the Mediterranean-style eating pattern," April 2019, https://www.diabetesfoodhub.org/articles/defining-the-mediterranean-diet.html

[10] "What is the Mediterranean diet? https://www.heart.org/en/healthy-living/healthy-eating/eat-smart/nutrition-basics/mediterranean-diet

[11] K. Gunnars and R. Link, "Mediterranean diet 101: A meal plan and beginner's guide," https:// www.healthline.com/nutrition/mediterranean-diet-meal-plan

[12] S. C. Degner et al., "Chapter 26 – Health benefits of traditional culinary and medicinal Mediterranean plants," *Complementary and Alternative Therapies and the Aging Population*, 2009, pp. 541-562.

[13] J. Leech, "The Nordic diet: An evidence-based review," February 2019, https://www.healthline.com/nutrition/the-nordic-diet-review#benefits

[14] M. Artemis, "Mediterranean diet," https://drartemis.com/diet-and-nutrition-guides/mediterranean-diet/#:~:text=Artemis%20is%20researching%20the%20Traditional,the%20University%20of%20Lancaster%2C%20UK.

[15] C. Obon et al., "A comparison study on traditional mixtures of herbal teas used in Eastern Mediterranean area," *Frontiers in Pharmacology,* vol. 12, April 2021.

[16] A. Djahafi, K. Taïbi, and L. A. Abderrahim, "Aromatic and medicinal plants used in traditional medicine in the region of Tiaret, North West of Algeria," *Mediterranean Botany*, vol. 42, 2921.

[17] C. Khatib, A. Nattouf, and M. I.H. Agha, "Traditional medicines used as adjuvant therapy for COVID-19 symptoms in Syria: An ethno-medicine survey" https://assets.researchsquare.com/files/rs-337854/v1/64327525-cd34-4b75-be75-0df398e861d1.pdf?c=1631879719

[18] E. Yegilada et al., "Traditional medicine in Turkey IV. Folk medicine in the Mediterranean subdivision," *Journal of Ethnopharmacology*, vol. 39, 1993, pp. 3 1-38.

[19] E. L. Unal et al., "Antimicrobial and antioxidant activities of some plants used as remedies in Turkish traditional medicine," *Pharmaceutical Biology*, vol. 46, no. 3, 2008, pp. 207-224.

[20] S. Lindberg, "Why the Mediterranean diet is touted as one of the best by dietitians," September 2020, https://www.businessinsider.in/science/health/news/why-the-mediterranean-diet-is-touted-as-one-of-the-best-by-dietitians/articleshow/78197425.cms#:~:text=Why%20the%20Mediterranean%20diet%20is%20touted%20as%20one%20of%20the%20best%20by%20dietitians,-Advertisement&text=The%20Mediterranean%20diet%20is%20a,chronic%20disease%20and%20overall%20mortality.

[21] "What is the best diet for osteoarthritis?" https://www.medicalnewstoday.com/articles/322603

[22] "Close adherence to traditional Mediterranean diet promotes longevity," June 2003, https://news.harvard.edu/gazette/story/2003/06/close-adherence-to-traditional-mediterranean-diet-promotes-longevity/

[23] F. J. Basterra-Gortari et al., "Effects of a Mediterranean eating plan on the need for glucose lowering medications in participants with type 2 diabetes: A Subgroup analysis of the PREDIMED trial diabetes," *Diabetes Care*, vol. 42, 2019, pp. 1390–1397.

[24] "Mediterranean diet meal plan for weight loss," https://www.mediterraneanliving.com/mediterranean-diet-meal-plan-for-weight-loss/

[25] M. Guasch-Ferré and W. C. Willett, "The Mediterranean diet and health: A comprehensive overview," *Journal of Internal Medicine,* vol. 290, no. 3, September 2021, pp. 549-566.

[26] K. Tsoutsoulopoulou, "Eating healthy and Mediterranean during pregnancy," https://www.samarasfoods.gr/en/livebetter/nutrition/eating-healthy-and-mediterranean-during-pregnancy

[28] "Our guide to the Mediterranean diet,"
https://www.medicalnewstoday.com/articles/324221

[29] "What actually is the Mediterranean diet,"
https://www.theguardian.com/society/2016/sep/02/mediterranean-diet-obesity-health-way-of-eating

[30] D. Robson, "Positive effects of the Mediterranean diet in the prevention and management of cardiovascular disease: A literature review," *Journal of the Australian Traditional-Medicine Society,* September 2014.

[31] H. Azaizeh et al., "The state of the art of traditional Arab herbal medicine in the Eastern region of the Mediterranean: A review," *Evidence-Based Complementary and Alternative Medicine,* vol. 3, no. 2, June 2006, pp. 229–235.

[32] G. L. Russo et al., "The Mediterranean diet from past to future: Key concepts from the second 'Ancel Keys' International Seminar," *Nutrition, Metabolism & Cardiovascular Diseases,* vol. 31, 2021, pp. 712-732.

[33] J. Mcdaniel and M. Taylor, *Prevention Mediterranean Table: 100 Vibrant Recipes to Savor and Share for Lifelong Health: A Cookbook.* Rodale Books 2017.

[34] K. A. Tessmer and S. Green, *The Complete Idiot's Guide to The Mediterranean Diet: Indulge in This Healthy, Balanced, Flavored Approach to Eating.* Alpha, 2010.

[35] C. Patorniti, *The 14 Day Mediterranean Diet Plan for Beginners: 100 Recipes to Kick-Start Your Health Goals.* Rockridge Press, 2020.

[36] Delightfulines Cookbooks, *The Convenient Mediterranean Diet Cookbook: A Simple Cookbook for Beginners with 100 Recipes, Full Color Pictures, and a Complete 30-Day Meal Plan.* Rockridge Press, 2020.

[37] A. Gellman, *The Mediterranean DASH Diet Cookbook: Lower Your Blood Pressure and Improve Your Health.* Rockridge Press, 2019.

[38] V. R. Preedy and R. R. Watson (eds.), *The Mediterranean Diet: An Evidence-Based Approach.* Academic Press, 2014.

[39] I. Lazarou, *Healthy Mediterranean Recipes with Medical Marijuana (CBD oil).* Independently Published, 2019.

[40] Z. Amar and E. Lev, *Arabian Drugs in Early Medieval Mediterranean Medicine. Edinburgh Studies in Classical Islamic History and Culture.* Edinburgh: Edinburgh University Press

[41] World Health Organization. *National Policy on Traditional Medicine and Regulation of Herbal Medicines: Report of a WHO Global Survey.* World Health Organization, 2005.

[42] E. Lev, *Practical Materia Medica of the Medieval Eastern Mediterranean According to the Cairo Genizah.* Brill, 2007.

[43] A. V. Arsdall and T. Graham (eds.), *Herbs and Healers from the Ancient Mediterranean through the Medieval West: Essays in Honor of John M. Riddle (Medicine in the Medieval Mediterranean).* Routledge, 2017.

[44] C. Savona-Ventura, *Traditional Medicine in a Mediterranean Island Community.* Lulu.com, 2021.

[45] R. Berman, *Mediterranean Diet For Dummies.* For Dummies, 2013.

[46] V. Harris, *1000 Mediterranean Meals: Every Recipe You Need for the Healthiest Way to Eat (Volume 1).* Chartwell Books, 2020.

[47] J. J. B. Anderson, *The Mediterranean Way of Eating.* Routledge, 2015.

[48] America's Test Kitchen, *The Complete Mediterranean Cookbook: 500 Vibrant, Kitchen-Tested Recipes for Living and Eating Well Every Day (The Complete ATK Cookbook Series).* America's Test Kitchen, 2016.

[49] M. Janes, *Mediterranean Diet Cookbook for Beginners: 1200-Day Quick & Easy Flavorful Recipes and 30-Day Meal Plan to Help You Burn Fat and Build Healthy Habits.* Independently Published, 2021.

[50] A. Riolo, *The Mediterranean Diabetes Cookbook.* American Diabetes Association, 2nd edition, 2019.

CHAPTER

Future of Traditional Medicine

"There is a great future for TCM if we can understand its fundamental principles."
—Mu-ming Poo

12.1 INTRODUCTION

Human history is essentially the history of medicines used to treat and prevent various diseases. Medicine has made a tremendous progress within the last 100 years. As different as our world is to that of our ancestors, we are still afflicted with many of the same ailments. The use of herbal medicines in the treatment of various diseases is as old as mankind. Our life and survival would have been impossible without the use of plant products.

As lofty profession as medicine is, it has not always gotten it right. Some practices that were once seen as controversial (such tradition medicines) is now standard of care. It is common to hear concerns about pharmaceutical companies marketing their products and influencing physicians [1]. Natural products from plants, animals, and minerals have been the basis of the treatment of human disease. A large portion of modern medicines worldwide are derived from natural products.

Tradition medicine (TM) refers to the combination of indigenous practices of medicine and several therapeutic experiences of many previous generations for the treatment, control, and management of illnesses. It entails health practices, approaches, knowledge, and beliefs incorporating plant, animal, and mineral based medicines, spiritual therapies, manual techniques, diagnose, and preventing illnesses or maintaining well-being. Today, traditional medicines are in demand and their popularity is increasing daily. They have been used to treat cut wounds, skin infection, swelling, aging, mental illness, cancer, asthma, diabetes, jaundice, scabies, venereal diseases, snakebite, and ulcer [2-4].

Western medicine is more common today. The traditional Chinese medicine (TCM) is a good example of a popular traditional medicine. A distinction is made between Chinese and Western medicine. The two medical practices can exist side by side. TCM's roots lie in 1st millennium BC. TCM covers five main areas: acupuncture, massage, plants and herbs, dietary therapy, and qigong exercises. The most widely known form of TCM treatment is acupuncture, shown in Figure 12.1, which has become part of Western medical healthcare practices [5]. China continues to attract a large number of foreigners annually. It still holds a mystic charm to the West. At its heart sits traditional Chinese medicine (TCM), which continues to hold the world's fascination as nations around the world try to grapple with the burdens of providing healthcare for ever-growing populations. Many Chinese doctors are often reluctant to use Chinese medicine because it is not lucrative. Although many Western doctors still regard TCM with suspicion, the World Health Organization officially recognize TCM in its global compendium [6]. The Chinese government works towards the survival of TCM and plans for the mutual learning and integration with Western medicine [7].

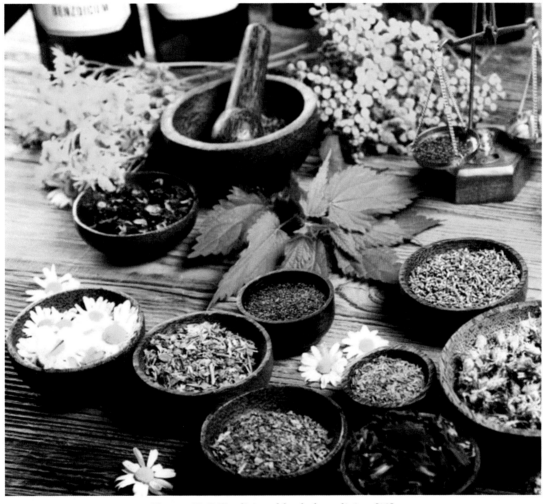

Figure 12.2 Traditional herbal medicine [10].

This chapter addresses the possible futures of traditional herbal medicines. It begins with the future of herbs in particular and the future of traditional medicine in general.

It highlights the benefits and challenges of traditional medicine. It addresses the globalization of traditional medicine. It also discusses the impact of emerging technologies on TM. The last section concludes with comments.

12.2 FUTURE OF HERBS

Although prophecy fascinates human beings, it has not been the fundamental goal of most medical figures who have talked about the future. In the past, medical writers invoked the future of medicine regularly and they often tended to take prediction lightly. As the history of medicine goes, forecasts can turn out to be correct or wrong [8].

Herbal medicines are the result of experiences of generations of practicing physicians of indigenous medicines for over hundreds of years. They refer to using a plant's seeds, berries, roots, leaves, bark, or flowers for medicinal purposes. Today, herbal medicines are in great demand in the developing world for primary healthcare. The use of herbal remedies throughout the world exceeds that of the conventional medicines by two to three times. The number of patients seeking alternate and herbal therapy is growing exponentially [9]. Statistics have revealed that about four billion people worldwide rely on plants or herbs as source of treatment. Herbal remedies have been used around the world for centuries to prevent and treat diseases. The increasing popularity of herbal medicine in recent times is due to the belief that all natural products are safe, cheaper, and easily available. Research efforts have been made in both developed and developing nations to scientifically evaluate and validate the herbal medicines. Figure 12.2 shows some herbal medicine [10].

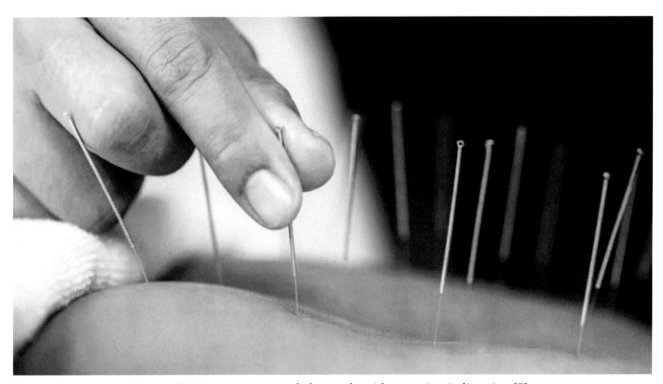

Figure 12.1 Acupuncture can help people with recurring indigestion [5].

The global herbal medicine market continues to grow on account of the increasing popularity of herbal products in developed nations. It is segmented based on product type, application, and geography. Based on product type, the market is divided into medicinal part, medicine function, and active ingredient. Based on application, the market is classified into traditional Chinese medicine, Indian traditional medicine, African traditional medicine, and many others. By geography, it is analyzed across North America, Europe, Asia-Pacific, and LAMEA [11]. Workers packing medical herbs for patients at a hospital in China are shown in Figure 12.3 [12].

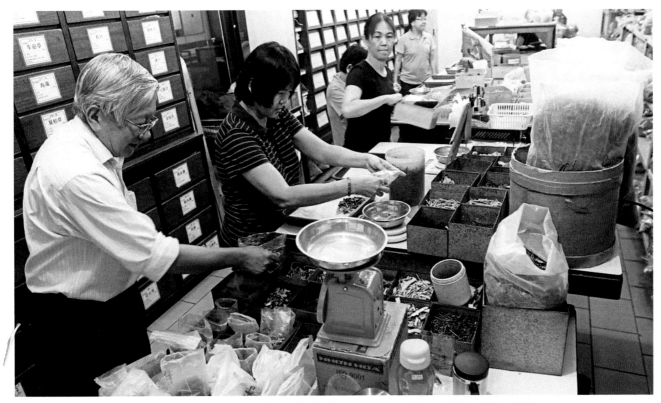

Figure 12.3 Workers packing herbs for patients at a hospital in China [12].

The herbal medicine is becoming more mainstream as there is improvements in the value of herbal medicine in the treating and preventing disease. The future of herbal medicine is inevitable integration of tradition and modern medical practices. This trend has been noticed by the World Health Organization (WHO). It can be achieved only when there is strong collaboration between government and all the actors in healthcare industry. The national governments should also institute pharmacovigilance unit for herbal medicine just like for conventional medicines. All the stakeholders must invest in research and development in order to properly integrate herbal medicine with conventional medicine [13]. Figure 12.4 illustrates the future prospects of herbal medicine.

12.3 FUTURE OF TRADITIONAL MEDICINE

Although the main consumers of medicinal plants have been the local population, the field has started to attract a number of foreign researchers who have discovered the value and efficacy of the traditional medicine. This interest has increased over the years. Medicinal chemists, pharmacologists, and the pharmaceutical industry worldwide have also come to consider traditional medicine (man commonly-used species) as a source that can be used in the preparation of synthetic medicine. For example, with the help of globalization, traditional Chinese medicine (TCM) has been widely used outside the Chinese community. Renowned hospitals outside Asia Pacific, like Mayo Clinic in the USA and the University College London Hospitals in the UK, have set up departments specializing in alternative forms of medicine including TCM.

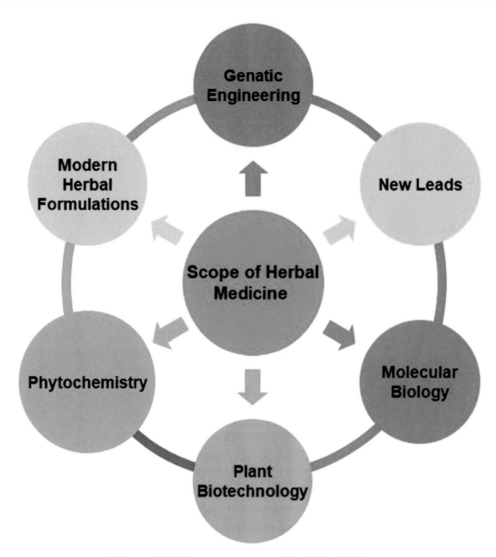

Figure 12.4 Future prospects of herbal medicine.

In recognition of the global importance of traditional medicine, the World Health Organization (WHO) has called for the incorporation of traditional medicine in public health services. The WHO is trying its best to facilitate the global standardization of the TM and herbal medicines. It recently announced that it will set up a Global Center for Traditional Medicine in India, which will become the center for global wellness. The center will strengthen the evidence, research, training, and awareness of traditional and complementary medicine [15].

The WHO's Traditional Medicine Program (TRM) has been responsible for promoting research and development of traditional, thereby impacting the healthcare of about four billion people worldwide. All 25 collaborating centers work together with the TRM to promote the safe and effective use of traditional medicines. The proper use of TM, its development, and its integration into national healthcare systems are in line with TRM. Such integration may be a means of expanding primary care in the modern health sector. In the future, traditional medicine will coexist with modern medicine. Medicinal plant research will depend on the development and the application of modern scientific methods, in the assessment of safety and efficacy [16]. Current academic institutions must include training qualified traditional medical doctors in every nation.

12.4 BENEFITS

TM is the oldest form of healthcare in the world and is used in the prevention and treatment of various illnesses. It has its own advantages and disadvantages in managing diseases. The TM market has grown at an expressive rate worldwide. This may be attributed to many important factors such as the belief that herbal drugs are free from side effects, safety of herbal medicines, and efficacy of herbal medicine in the treatment of some diseases where conventional therapies have proved to be inadequate. In order to address the problem of drug shortage or high cost, many health-oriented ministries are now encouraging the use of local medicinal plants for disease treatment.

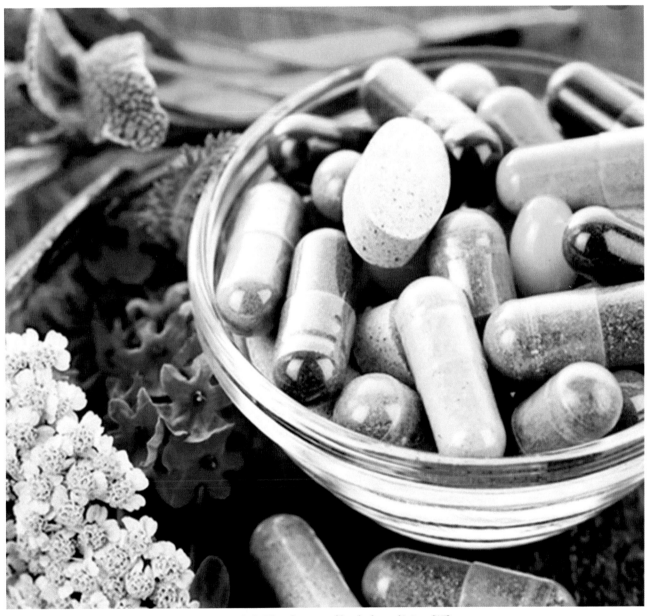

Figure12.5 The future of herbal medicine [17].

Currently, there are many companies are producing TM. Herbal medicine has a huge market potential in the future. The future of medicine delivery is online. Figure 12.5 illustrates the future of herbal medicine [17]. Other benefits include the following [18]:

- *Alternative Medicine:* The high cost of drugs and increase in drug resistance to common diseases like malaria has caused the therapeutic approach to alternative traditional medicine. Alternative medicine works better for just about everything else specially for chronic disease. TM provide us with new alternatives to synthetic drugs. It focuses on health maintenance and shows great advantages in early intervention, personalized, and combination therapies.

- *Efficacy:* Majority of the rural people and the urban poor rely on the use of herbal medicine when they are ill. There can be no doubt about the acceptability and efficacy of herbal remedy within African communities. Traditional healing is flourishing in urban settings where the Western is either not available or expensive.

- *Inadequacy in Western Healthcare:* In Western medical treatment, treatment is divorced from the patient's culture. The treatment only addresses a patient's biological manifestation of the illness and does not attempt to heal spiritual aspects of illness. The traditional medicine avoids all of this and is free from side effects. Herbal medicine is preferred in the treatment of certain diseases where conventional medicines have proven to be inadequate.

- *Holistic Treatment:* Holism is one of the basic characteristics and a major advantage of TM. TM maintains that the human body is an organic whole and inseparable from the external natural surroundings. Traditional medical treatment is holistic or whole-body. The TM system relies on the delicate balance between the mind, body, and spirit. TM pays attention to the whole and individual parts of the body. It uses a unique holistic approach to cure human diseases through establishment of equilibrium in the human life, body, mind, intellect, and soul.

- *Medical Significance:* TM is well known for being accessible, available, acceptable, dependable, and compatible with the human body, with minimal side effects. It plays a huge role in large population of infectious patients. Many TM products are widely utilized as anti-diabetic agents and anti-cancer drugs worldwide. These kinds of drugs play key roles in the treatment of various diseases. TM works better for just about illness, specially for chronic disease.

- *High Cost:* Modern healthcare services provided by hospitals are expensive relation to the income of the rural population. In view of the high cost, governments are now encouraging the use of local medicinal plants for disease treatment.

- *Pharmaceutical Industry:* The pharmaceutical industry now considers using traditional medicine in the preparation of synthetic medicine. Some of necessary medicinal plant species are available and used around the world.

- *Infections:* An area where traditional medicines can offer hope is in the treatment of infections. There are a number of plants that offer solutions for the treatment of bacterial, fungal, viral, protozoa, HIV, and other opportunistic infections.

These benefits are illustrated in Figure 12.6.

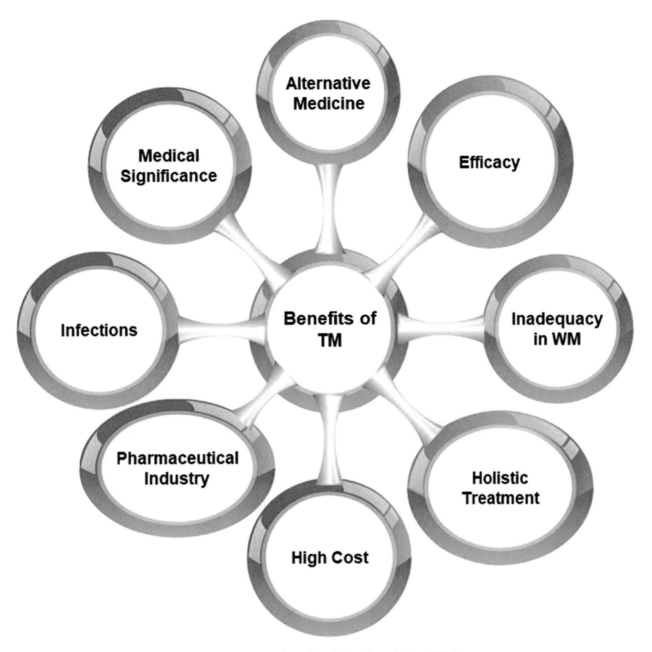

Figure 12.6 Benefits of traditional medicine (TM).

12.5 CHALLENGES

It is difficult to deny the limitations of traditional medicine, which include improper dosage, low hygiene standards, and the secrecy of some healing methods. To reach a stage where herbal medicine becomes integrated into conventional treatment, some issues have to be addressed.

Other challenges include the following [18–21].

- *Insufficient Documentation:* There insufficient documentation and scientific experimentation for verification of the herbalist's claims. For most of the traditional practices, information about efficacy, safety, and quality is poor. Written records about the patients are absent.

- *Loss of Indigenous Knowledge:* Traditional medical knowledge is often passed on orally from generation to generation, in some cases with families specializing in specific treatments. In some countries, medicinal plants are on the verge of total disappearance. Loss of indigenous knowledge on their medicinal potential is also fast increasing. This may continue until the younger generations are adequately educated about the importance of traditional medicine in our society and its major role in restoring health.

- *Healthcare in Rural Areas:* The lack of healthcare systems in rural areas leads to inadequate technical services and poor quality care. This often compels local people to treat themselves using medicinal herbs before going to a traditional practitioner or a modern doctor.

- *No Political Will:* There is a lack of political will among political leaders to support the research and development of local medicines. There is also a lack of institutional support for production and dissemination of key species. This leads to a lack of state-of-the-art equipment to promote R&D, quality control, and quality assurance of traditional medicine. For example, although herbals drugs from Ayurveda are gaining popularity, no injectable Ayurvedic drug is available to manage the acute diseases at the moment. Therefore, researchers should intensity effort for developing standardized drugs.

- *Skepticism:* A major challenge is skepticism is in the developing world, particularly the youths who are more familiar with Western medicine.

- *Slow Collaboration:* There has been a slow collaboration between modern medical doctors and traditional medicine practitioners. This is possibly due to lack of legal framework and official recognition of TM by conventional medicine. Herbal medicine and modern medicine are interrelated for practical values. Integrating them should be a top priority. Herbal medicines need to be translated into modern drug developments and clinical evaluations.

- *Interaction:* The problem of drug-herbal interaction is an important issue. Some patients often use traditional and conventional medicines together. The interaction of these two types of medications may be dangerous. It has raised serious concern about the safety of the patients. There are case reports of serious adverse events after administration of herbal products along with modern medicine. Patients should consult their doctor before taking both drugs.

- *Quality Control:* While traditional herbal products are heterogeneous, they contain several challenges to qualify control, and the regulatory process. There are currently many herbal products on the market and the quality control of these products is of paramount importance. Quality control of herbal extracts and finished products is usually carried out using a series of clinical trials that met international quality standards.

- *Intellectual Property:* Some indigenous researchers publish their works without protecting them. The protection of intellectual property rights should be extended to traditional medicine. Loss of indigenous knowledge on TM is fast increasing and this may continue until the younger generations are adequately enlightened about the importance of TM.

- *Ethics:* There is lack of the code of conduct in the practice of TM. This has led to abuse of significant magnitude. Herbal products are sold with poor labeling and without instruction. They are also sold without any scientific studies on their safety. There is lack of documentation on medicinal plants and lack of control over what is the market for consumption.

- *Deforestation:* There are roughly 250,000 species in the world, with only a relatively small proportion of them are used for their medicinal properties, with both medical and economic consequences. Although medical herbs are a major source for new drug discovery, a great number of them may likely go into extinction, majorly due to deforestation. In fact, deforestation poses a clear threat to the future of herbal medicines. There is a threat of extinction to certain species of plants. High demand of TM now appears to be endangering supply.

Some of these challenges are shown in Figure 12.7.

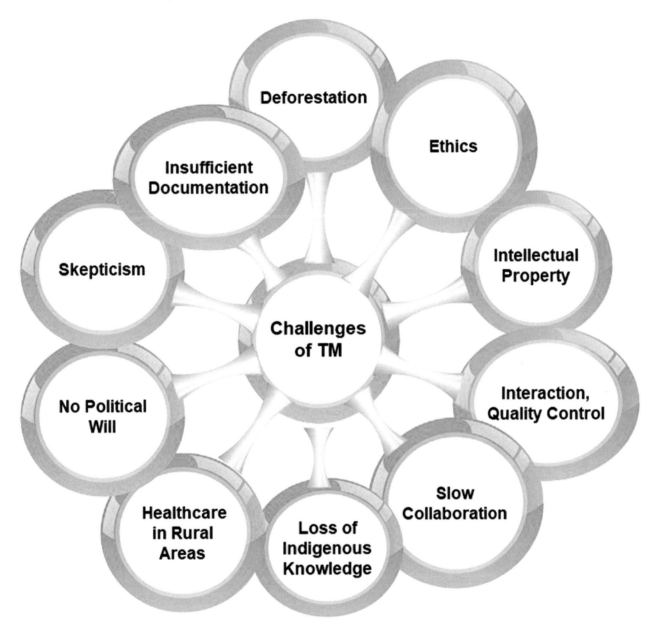

Figure 12.7 Challenges of traditional medicine.

12.6 GLOBALIZATION OF TRADITIONAL MEDICINE

An urgent global need is to find an effective and economic way to overcome all ailments of humanity. This will require integrating traditional medicine and Western medicine together. While modern medicine is aimed at suppressing symptoms in one isolated area, traditional medicine attempts to identify and restore the underlying imbalance of the body. Their marriage is important for the future of medicine, but achieving this is an uphill task. The World Health Organization (WHO) has called for the integration of traditional medicine in public health services. Through modernization, collaboration, organization, and integration, traditional medicine may be an expedient way of expanding primary care in the modern health sector. The organization of traditional medicine practice will bring about a controlled practice and harmonized team of traditional medical practitioners. Their integration into the national health sector is the only way to move forward. It forms the basis for the medicine of the future [21]. TM should go through robust experimental and clinical verification. Researchers, manufacturers, and regulatory agencies should carry out intense scientific studies and clinical trials on TM. This way, all criticisms against TM can be chipped away to make it acceptable in mainstream healthcare.

Traditional medicine occupies a significant place in healthcare system around the world. It promises a way to a more balanced life in stressful times. The consumption of medicinal plant has caused an increasing practice in herbal medicines (including Ayurveda, Chinese traditional medicines, and alternative therapies). Today, the world is growing up with complementary medicine due to vast benefits for life long. The traditional medicines now coexist and complement Western medicine throughout Africa, Asia, Latin America, and the Middle East. The future of traditional medicine is not just convenient, affordable, and available, but designed around the customers' needs.

If the World Health Organization intends to provide healthcare for all, some positive steps need to be taken to develop traditional medicine. TM should be allowed to thrive and establish an independent and competitive educational system for TM doctors, equivalent to Western medicine. It is important for each nation or ethnic group to compile an encyclopedia of medicinal plants used in traditional medicine.

Not everybody is happy with the modernization and globalization of TM. Some in the medical community claim WHO overlooked the potential toxicity of some herbal medicine, poor diagnosis, unknown efficacy, and lack of evidence that TM works. They are concerned that TM will jeopardize the health of unsuspecting consumers worldwide. Some animal rights advocates claim it will further endanger animals such as the tiger, pangolin, bear, and rhino, whose organs are used in some TCM cures [22].

12.7 MODERN TECHNOLOGIES

Today, information technology has infiltrated all walks of life, and tradition medicine is no exception. A closer scientific look at TM using modern technologies should be in the interest of the patients, physicians, and other stakeholders. In order to break through the fierce competition, traditional medicine practitioners must learn to flexibly use modern, emerging technologies such as big data, artificial intelligence, and data mining [24-26]:

- *Artificial Intelligence*: In the field of Chinese medicine, as early as the 1980s, Chinese scholars started the initial attempt to combine traditional Chinese medicine and artificial intelligence. Artificial intelligence refers to intelligence demonstrated by machines, while the natural intelligence is the intelligence displayed by humans and animals. The use of artificial intelligence–related technologies to learn and simulate the clinical experience of old and famous traditional Chinese medicine to diagnose the patient will have a very important clinical significance for Chinese medicine.
- *Data Mining:* Data mining is the task of discovering useful patterns from a large amount of data. It is recognized as a rapidly emerging research area. Data mining has found application in nearly

all the TM areas. Technically, it serves as a support for the TM modernization process. It is clear-crystal that the information plays a critical role in the TM. We presently face with an ever-increasing volume of medical data and different treatment approaches taken in the TM. the data normalization and medical ontology development might prove to be effective in attaining higher levels of recognition and information technology application in TM.

- *Big Data:* Big data refers to a collection of data that cannot be captured, managed, and processed by conventional software tools. Big data analytics is a modern technology that can help make traditional medical practices "evidence based" by unveiling previously "invisible" information about their efficacy, interactions, and effects.

12.8 CONCLUSION

Traditional medical systems now coexist and complement Western medicine throughout Africa, Asia, and Latin America. Traditional medicine needs to be officially legalized and made part of the mainstream healthcare system in every country. The prospects for doing this are quite high. Although the future may seem oblique for the amalgamation of both the modern and traditional medicine, it is a win–win situation. The integration of traditional medicine and modern practice will bring about a controlled practice, more responsible, and well harmonized medicine and collaboration among healthcare practitioners.

The safety, efficacy, and effectiveness of TM are still controversial in China and the rest of the world. The global market for traditional medicine is expected to grow. The future of traditional medicine is bright. More information on the future of TM can be found in the books in [16,27,28] and the following related journals:

- *Journal of Herbal Medicine*
- *Journal of Medicinal Plants Studies*
- *Journal of Ethnopharmacology*
- *Journal Herbmed Pharmacology*
- *Journal of Ethnobiology and Ethnomedicine*
- *Journal of Traditional Medicine & Clinical Naturopathy*
- *Chinese Journal of Integrative Medicine*
- *The Development of Nutraceuticals and Traditional Medicine*
- *African Journal of Traditional, Complementary and Alternative Medicine*
- *Current Traditional Medicine*
- *International Journal of Traditional Medicine and Applications*

REFERENCES

[1]   S. Roberts, "The future of medicine: A brief history of alternative medicine and my hope for the future,"
https://www.phopkinsmd.com/the-future-of-medicine/

[2]   S. Verma and S. P. Singh, "Current and future status of herbal medicines," *Veterinary World,* vol.1, no. 11, November 2008, pp. 347-350.

[3]   M. S. A. Khan and I. Ahmad, "Chapter 1 - Herbal medicine: Current trends and future prospects," *New Look to Phytomedicine*, 2019, pp. 3-13.

[4]   M. N. O. Sadiku, U. C. Chukwu, A. Ajayi-Majebi, S. M. Musa, "Future of traditional medicine," *International Journal of Trend in Scientific Research and Development,* vol. 6, no. 1, November-December 2021, pp.1301-1307.

[5]   B. Curley, "Acupuncture may be effective at reducing indigestion symptoms," May 2020, https://www.healthline.com/health-news/acupuncture-effective-reducing-indigestion-symptoms

[6]   M. A. Karanja, "Is traditional Chinese medicine the future of global healthcare?" June 2020, https://www.beijing-kids.com/blog/2020/06/06/traditional-chinese-medicine-future-global-healthcare-differences-tcm-western-medicine/

[7]   C. Abbey, "New law sparks debate over future of traditional Chinese medicine," June 2017, https://www.cnn.com/2017/06/29/health/china-new-law-traditional-chinese-medicine-tcm/index.html

[8]   J. C. Burnham, "Presidential address: The past of the future of medicine," *Bulletin of the History of Medicine,* vol. 67, no. 1, Spring 1993, pp. 1-27.

[9]   S. K. Pal and Y. Shukla, "Herbal medicine: Current status and the future," *Asian Pacific Journal of Cancer Prevention,* vol. 4, no. 4, August-December, 2003, pp. 281-288.

[10]   "Is the future of medicine rooted in the past?" February 2019, https://sites.psu.edu/globalhealthissues/2019/02/06/is-the-future-of-medicine-rooted-in-the-past/

[11]   "Herbal medicine demand and trends 2024," http://www.rnrmarketresearch.com/contacts/request-sample?rname=1937471

[12]   L. J. Xian, " Future of traditional Chinese medicine," November 2020, Unknown Source.

[13]   Y. O. Ahmed, "Herbal medicine: Past, present and future," June 2019, https://www.researchgate.net/publication/333868025_HERBAL_MEDICINE_PAST_PRESENT_AND_FUTURE

[15]   Taboola, "WHO to set up global centre on traditional medicine in India: PM Modi," November 2020, https://www.ndtv.com/india-news/who-to-set-up-global-centre-on-traditional-medicine-in-india-says-pm-modi-2324771

[16]   G. B. Mahady, "World health and international collaboration in traditional medicine and medicinal plant research," in D. Eskinazi (ed.), *What Will Influence the Future of Alternative Medicine? A World Perspective.* World Scientific, 2011, pp.89-103.

[17]   Northlines, "Future of herbal medicine," September 2020, https://www.thenorthlines.com/future-of-herbal-medicine/

[18]   C. N. Fokunang, "Traditional medicine: Past, present and future research and development prospects and integration in the national health system of Cameroon," *African Journal of Traditional, Complementary and Alternative Medicine,* vol. 8, no. 3, 2011, pp. 284–295.

[19]   R. Mirzaeian et al., "Progresses and challenges in the traditional medicine information system: A systematic review," *Journal of Pharmacy & Pharmacognosy Research,* vol. 7, no. 4, 2019, pp. 246-259.

[20]   E. C. Chukwuma, M. O. Soladoye, and R. T. Feyisola, "Traditional medicine and the future of medicinal plants in Nigeria," *Journal of Medicinal Plants Studies,* vol. 3, no. 4, 2015, pp. 23-29.

[21]   "The future of medicine," February 2019, https://www.krithika.net/the-future-of-medicine/

[22]   "Herbal medicine: Current status and the future," November 2018,

https://qs-gen.com/herbal-medicine-current-status-and-the-future-2/

[23] K. Hunt, "Chinese medicine gains WHO acceptance but it has many critics," May 2019, https://www.cnn.com/2019/05/24/health/traditional-chinese-medicine-who-controversy-intl/index.html

[24] M. Mukerji and M. Sagner, "Genomics and big data analytics in Ayurvedic medicine," *Progress in Preventive Medicine,* vol. 4, no. 1, April 2019.

[25] J. Liu et al., "The future development of traditional Chinese medicine from the perspective of artificial intelligence with big data," *Proceedings of the 4th IEEE International Conference on Big Data Security on Cloud*, 2018, pp. 204-209.

[26] M. N. O. Sadiku, *Emerging Internet-Based Technologies.* Boca Raton, FL: CRC Press, 2019.

[27] F. Murad, A. Rahman, and Ka Bian, *Herbal Medicine: Back to the Future: Volume 1, Vascular Health.* Bentham Science Publishers, 2019.

[28] P. K. Mukherjee (eds.), *Traditional Medicine and Globalization- The Future of Ancient Systems of Medicine.* Kolkata, India: Maven Publishers, 2014.

APPENDIX A

Other Topics

This appendix is a list of other traditional medicines that are not covered in this book.

1. Australian Traditional Medicine
2. Brazilian Traditional Medicine
3. Caribbean Traditional Medicine
4. Ethiopian Traditional Medications
5. Greek Classic/Ancient Medicine
6. Jamaican Traditional Medicine
7. Jordanian Traditional Medicine
8. Korean Traditional Medicine
9. Malay Traditional Medicine
10. Russian Traditional Medicine
11. Thai Traditional Medicine
12. Tibetan Traditional Medicine
13. Traditional Aborginal Medicine
14. Traditional Bumese Medicine
15. Traditional Lau Medicine
16. Traditional Medicine in South Africa
17. Traditional Medicine in Sri Lanka
18. Traditional Nepalia Medicine
19. Traditional Oriental Medicine
20. Traditional Tibetan Medicine
21. Vietnamese Traditional Medicine

INDEX

A

Acupuncture, 24,26,56,62,67
Affordability, 94
Africa, 13,84,86,88
African medical practice, 86
African medicine, 91
African traditional medicine (ATM), 83,84,85,88,92-94,97
    Benefits of, 94
    Challenges of, 95,96
    History of, 84
    Regulation of, 91
Afrocentricity, 84
Ageing, 63,128
Allah (God), 136,138
Alligator pepper, 107
Aloe Vera, 43,107,141
Alternative medicine, 5,17,83
Alzheimer's disease (AD), 28,75
American Medical Association (AMA), 16
Anxiety, 157
Arabic herbal medicine, 8
Arabic scholar, 141
Arabic traditional medicine (ATM), 137,142,147
Arabic world, 8
Artificial intelligence, 194
Ashitaba plant, 60
Availability, 159
Ayurveda, 8,36-38,40,45,50
    Applications of, 44,45
    Benefits of, 47,48
    Challenges of, 48-50
    Diagnosis of, 40
    Globalization of, 45
    Specialties in, 42
    Treatment by, 41
    Wisdom of, 51

B

Basil, 168,169
Big data, 195
Bitter kola nuts, 107
Bitter leaf, 106

Black Africa, 84
Blood, 121
Brain health, 177

C

California College of Ayurveda (CCA), 51
California School of Herbal Studies, 162
Cancer, 28,45,64,128,143,157,174
Canon of Medicine, 120,121,139
Cardiovascular diseases, 13,127,175
China, 3,7,12,32,33
Chinese government, 23,30,185
Christianity, 84,90,101
Cilandro, 155,156
Colonialism, 84
Complementary and alternative medicine (CAM), 5,17
Complementary medicine, 5,16,17,83
Confucianism, 7
Constipation, 126
Coriander, 43
Coronavirus, 157, see also COVID-19
Cost, 64,158
Cost effectiveness, 111
COVID-19, 91,127,143
Culture Clash, 14,78,160
Curanderismo, 153

D

Data mining, 194
Deficiency, 25
Deforestation, 192
Dehydration, 143
Demons, 103
Depression, 92,126,157
Diabetes, 45,91,110,157,175,178
Diagnosis, 40
Diarrhea, 109,158
Diet of Algeria, 173
Diet of Crete, 173
Diet of Greece, 173
Diet of Syria, 174
Diet of Turkey, 174

Dietary supplements, 47
Disease prevention, 58
Diseases, 22,76,101,184
Divination, 86
Drug, 44
Dual healthcare system, 16

E

Ear Acupuncture, 75
East Africa, 90
Efficacy, 77,91,190
Egypt, 84
Epilepsy, 127
Erectile dysfunction (ED), 109
Ethics, 14,144,192
Europe, 80
European Commission, 17
European Herbal and Traditional Medicine Practitioners
     Association (EHTPA), 73
European Medicines Agency, 72
European traditional medicine (ETM), 71
     Applications of, 75
     Benefits of, 77
     Challenges, 77-79
     Globalization of, 76
European Union, 12,71,73
Evil spirits, 103
Extinction of plants, 49,145

F

Fasting, 143
Fever, 109,157
Folk medicine, 70,83,153
Food, 36

G

Garlic, 11
Ghana, 12,89
Ginger, 11,156
Ginkgo biloba,10,11
Global Acceptance, 47
Global Center for Traditional Medicine, 188
Globalization, 79,166
God, 84
Governments, 15
Gynaecology, 92

H

Headache, 126
Health, 1,54,101,134,138
Health conditions, 1

Healthcare, 20,189
     In rural areas, 192
Heart health, 177
Herbal medicines, 1,3,9,24-26,42,73,75,80,86,123,
     140,146,186,187,189
Herbal preparations, 76
Herbal products, 17
Herbal supplements, 12
Herbalist, 87
Herbs, 1,9,60
     Future of, 185
High blood pressure, 109,155
History of medicine, 3
Holistic medicine, 6,77
Holistic treatment, 65,94,144,190
Holy Quran, 134,136,139
Homeopathy, 39
Honey, 141
Human body, 22
Human history, 184

I

Ibn-Sina (Avicenna), 136,139
India, 12,36,41,42,44,50
Indian herbal medicines, 42
Infections, 190
Infertility, 127,144
Integration, 46,113,160
Integrative medicine, 4,65
Intellectual property, 192
Interaction, 159,192
Interference, 113
International Day of Yoga, 39
Iranian traditional medicine, 119,120
Islam, 101
Islamic medicine, 134
Islamic Republic of Iran, 129
Islamic traditional medicine, 137
Islamic world, 3

J

Japan, 7,54,55
Japanese acupuncture, 62
Japanese herbal medicine, 59
Japanese traditional medicine (JTM), 64,67
     Applications of, 61

K

Kampo, 7,54,57,59,67
     Applications of, 61
     Benefits of, 64,65
     Challenges of. 66

Characteristics of, 57
Diagnosis of, 58
History of, 55
Globalization of, 66
Pillars of, 56
Kampo practitioner, 67
Kola nut, 106
Korea, 7

L

Legislation, 160
Liver cleansing, 126
Longevity, 174,178
Low cost,13,47

M

Magic, 105
Malaria, 91,108
Marginalization, 159
Massage therapy, 62
Medicinal herbs, 105
Medicinal plants, 9,42,187
Medicine, 54,101,184
Medieval Islamic medicine, 134
Mediterranean diet, 167,169-180
Benefits of, 176-178
Challenges of, 179
Globalization of, 179
History of, 167
Mediterranean herbs, 168
Mediterranean medicine, 3
Mediterranean nations, 171
Mexican plants, 154
Mexican traditional health, 159
Mexican traditional medicine, 159
Benefits, 158
Challenges of, 159-161
Globalization of, 161
Mexico, 150-154,158,162
Middle East, 143,159
Modern medicine, 3,17,64
Modern technologies, 194
Modernization, 166
Muslim, 139
Muslim countries, 142
Muslim scholars, 134

N

Nigeria, 8,84,89,97,101,108
Nordic Diet, 173
Northern Nigeria, 142
Nutrition, 47

O

Obesity, 64,127,158,175
Oduduwa, 102
Olive oil, 140,171
Olodumare, 102
Onion, 141
Oogun, 104
Orunmila, 102
Osteoarthritis, 174
Overdose, 113
Overexploitation, 15
Overweight, 144,175

P

Peppermint, 156
People's Republic of China, 20
Persia, 120
Persian traditional medicine, 119,122,123,130
Applications, 126
Benefits of, 128
Challenges of, 129
Globalization of, 129
History of, 120
Persian traditional practitioners, 123
Pharmacology, 28
Philosophy, 29
Plagiarism, 49
Popular herbs, 10
Practitioners of traditional medicine, 9,14
Pregnancy, 175
Prophet Muhammad, 120,138,141

Q

Qatar, 142

R

Regulation, 14,49,66,78,113,145,160
Roots, 88
Rosemary, 157,168

S

Safety, 14,49,77,78,91,113,159
Saudi Arabia, 142
School of Persian Medicine, 129,130
Scientific evidence, 49
Scientific validation, 14
Scorpion poisoning, 158
Secrecy, 14,113
Shea butter, 89,106
Siddha, 38
Side effects, 49,64,66

Skepticism, 30
Sleeplessness, 126
South Africa, 8,84,89
Southwestern Nigeria, 104
Spiritual healing, 47
Spiritualism, 86
Standardization, 14,31,49
Stone Age, 86
Stroke, 109

T

Tongue diagnosis, 27
Toxicity, 31,49,66,78,113,145
Traditional African medicine, 8,92
Traditional African Medicine Day, 8
Traditional Arabic and Islamic medicine (TAIM), 136,147
    Benefits of, 144
    Challenges of, 145,146
    Globalization of, 146
Traditional Chinese medicine (TCM), 6,7,20,25,26,32,
    33,55,76,187
    Applications of, 26
    Benefits of, 29,30
    Challenges of, 30
    Five elements of, 22
    Four principles of, 23
    History of, 21
    Modernization of, 28
    Practitioners of, 24
    Standardization of, 31
Traditional East Asian Medicine (TEAM), 57
Traditional European medicine (TEM), 71,74
Traditional healers, 85,87
Traditional Indian medicine (TIM), 8,37,40,50
Traditional Japanese medicine,7,54,55
Traditional Knowledge Digital Library (TKDL), 16
Traditional Korean Medicine, 7
Traditional medical knowledge, 16
Traditional medical systems, 195
Traditional medication, 2-4
Traditional medicinal systems, 3
    around the world, 7
Traditional medicine, 2,6,16,17,36,70,83,101,103,194
    Benefits of, 13
    Categories of, 6,7
    Challenges of, 14,15
    Future of, 184
    Globalization of, 14,193
    Standardization of, 14
Traditional medicine practitioners, 14,105
Traditional Medicine Program (TRM), 188
Traditional Mediterranean diet (MedDiet), 166

Traditional Mexican healing/healer, 151,153
Traditional Mexican medicine (MTM), 151,152,163
    History of, 152
Trust, 47
Tuberculosis (TB), 158
Tubers, 88
Tzu Chi, 162

U

United Arab Emirates (UAE), 142
United States, 13,21,51
University of Traditional Medicine, 80

V

Vegetables, 170

W

Water therapy, 63
Weight loss, 177
Western medicine, 2-5,55,94,129,184,193
Whole grains, 170
Wisdom of life, 40
Woman infertility, 110
World Health Organization (WHO), 4,16,20,46,66,70,72,
    83,97,101,115,119,150,185,187,188,194
Worldwide Acceptance, 29

Y

Yokukansan (YKS), 57
Yoga, 36,39
Yoruba, 101
Yoruba traditional medicine (YTM), 102,105,115
    Benefits of, 111,112
    Challenges of, 112-114
    Globalization of, 115

Z

Zambia, 90
Zhang Gongyao, 21

Printed in the United States
by Baker & Taylor Publisher Services